Dr. Murad & Nitric Oxide

"Can increase your life expectancy with proper diet, exercise and nutritional supplements that increase NO production and effects"
1998 Nobel Prize winner in Physiology or Medicine, Dr. Ferid Murad.
by Ferid Murad, M.D. Ph.D., and
Daniel Cheng-Shing Chen, M.D. Ph.D.

The contents of this book are a reflection of the authors' philosophy, beliefs and clinical experience. The ideas, suggestions, and procedures presented in the book are not intended to be a substitute for consultation with your own physician before beginning any new regimen.

PUBLISHER: Daniel, Cheng-Shing, Chen M.D., Ph.D.
Address: No. 14, Wenchang E. 5th St., Beitun Dist., Taichung City 40666, Taiwan (R.O.C.)
Tel: +886-4-2236-6766, Fax: +886-4-2236-6386
E-mail: service@feridmuad.com.tw

ISBN-13: 9781492983187

My Life-long Endeavor

Dr. Ferid Murad, Physician and Doctor of Medicine

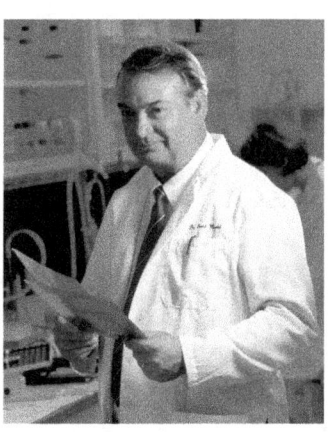

- Professor at George Washington University.
- Inventor behind the theory of the wellknown drug "Viagra".
- Winner of the American Heart Association Ciba Award in 1988.
- Winner of the Albert and Mary Lasker Award for Basic Research in 1996.
- Member of the U.S. National Academy of Sciences since 1997.
- 1998 Nobel Prize Winner in Physiology or Medicine. Member of the U.S. Institute of Medicine since 1998.
- Winner of the Baxter award for Distinguished Research in the Biomedical Sciences in 2000.
- Foreign Member of the Chinese Academy of Sciences since 2007.

Dr. Murad has also collaborated on over 440 highly acclaimed medical publications.

Dr. Murad was born in 1936 in a small room above a baker's shop in the U.S. state of Indiana. From a young age he washed plates and waited tables in the family restaurant to help raise money for school fees. Dr. Murad has fond memories of these times; "I would wait on customers and not record what they had ordered or how much it had cost. I would then tally up the price in my head. This proved to be great practice for my future career in scientific research".

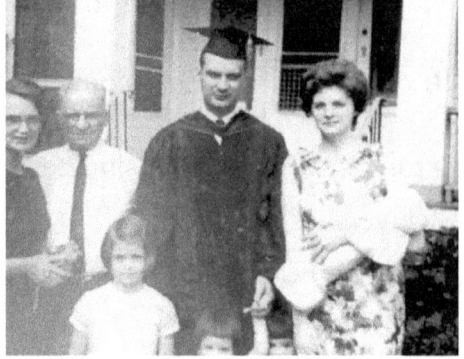

Dr. Murad (second from right) with his wife (far right), parents and kids in 1965.

Dr. Murad describes how his parents had a strong influence on both his and his two brothers' educational and career choices. His parents placed great importance on education, but it was from his mother and grandmother that he learned about compassion and generosity, which ultimately influenced him to choose medicine.

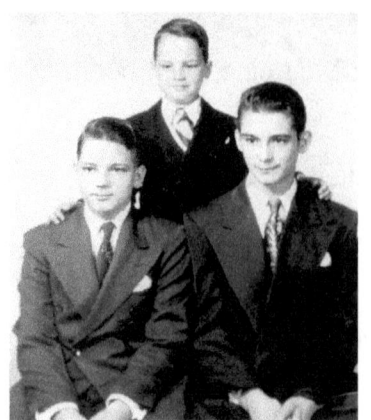

Dr. Murad (right) and his brothers at a young age.

Dr. Murad employs both clinical and pharmacological approaches to treat patients suffering from all kinds of physical illness. As a sixth grade student, Dr. Murad made an important decision about his future career path by establishing three main career objectives: to become a doctor, a teacher and a pharmacologist. Nowadays he does all these. Yet what helped fuel this determination? Dr. Murad believes that his teachers greatly encouraged him, and he has always had a strong personal desire to leave a mark on society through his contributions to scientific development.

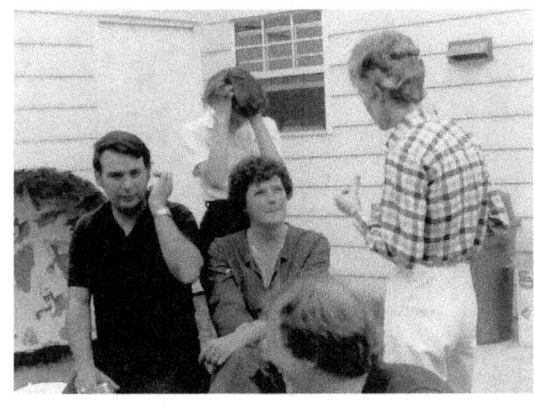

Dr. Murad (far left) with his wife Carol (center) and lab colleagues in 1980.

When Dr. Murad first revealed to his parents that he had decided to go into medical research, his parents were somewhat disappointed. They believed that he could earn more money practicing as a doctor. "Yet I knew that if I was lucky with my research, then there would be no end to the amount of people I could help." Glancing at those others in the room, Dr. Murad explained how he hoped that he could help many more people to live healthier and happier lives. He proudly admits that he is very lucky to have such a wonderful family, with 5 kids and 9 grandchildren, but that his career will always take precedence.

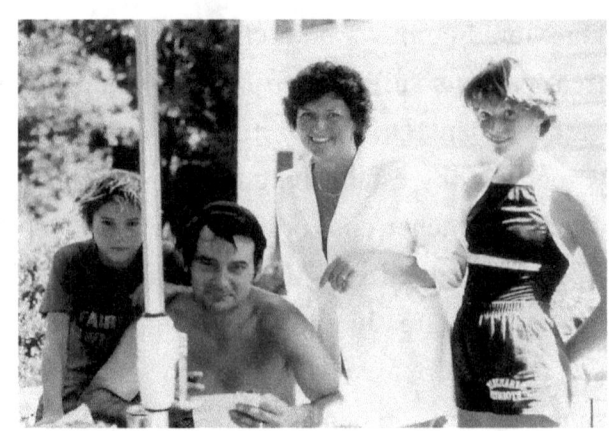

Dr. Murad (second left) with his wife Carol (second right) and two of his children in 1978.

Lasker Medical Research Award

—— A marker for the Nobel Prize

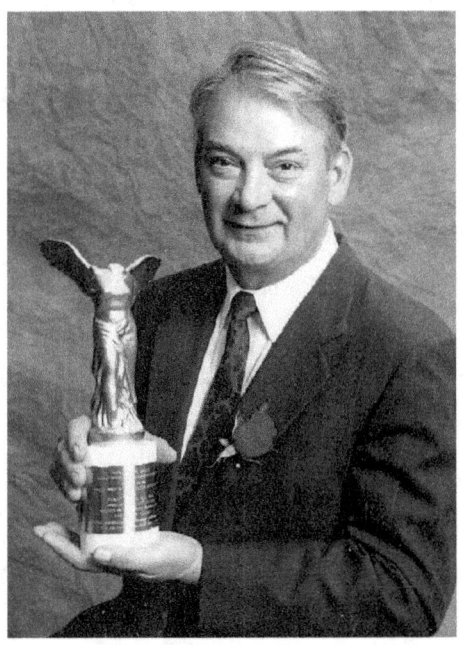

In 1996 Dr. Murad received the Albert and Mary Lasker Award for Basic Medical Research.

The 1996 Albert and Mary Lasker Award for Basic Medical Research.

Dr. Murad has received many awards and honors. In addition to the acclaimed Nobel Prize, he also won the Lasker Award, known informally as "America's Nobel". In 1996, Dr. Murad received the Lasker Award for Basic Medical Research.

The Lasker Medical Award, which recognizes outstanding

contributions in the medical profession, is America's most prestigious biomedical award.

The Lasker was originally set up as three separate awards: Basic Medical Research, Clinical Medical Research and Public Service. in the year 2000, it was renamed the Mary Woodard Lasker Award, in honor of Mrs. Lasker. In 2007, an additional special contribution award was added, known as the Special Achievement Award.

In September of each year, the Lasker Foundation will announce the winners at the end of the month. At the awards ceremony, the winners will receive a prize, and will be awarded a statuette of the Winged Victory of Samothrace with their name engraved on this symbol of victory over disease and death.

The shortlist for the Lasker Award is usually announced in September, while the Nobel Prize is usually announced in October. Moreover, many of the winners of the basic medical research award have gone on to receive the Nobel Prize. Since 1962, more than half of those scientists who received the Lasker Award, also won the Nobel Prize. To date, over 300 people have received the Lasker Award, and at least 83 of these people have won the Nobel Prize. So the Lasker Award in the medical profession has been nicknamed the "Nobel Prize marker." 1996 Lasker Award was a great accomplishment for Dr. Murad, and established him as an extremely influential scientist. Therefore in 1998 when he was awarded the Nobel Prize, in the eyes of the world, Dr. Murad undeniably deserved it.

The highest honor - The Nobel Prize

In 1998, Dr. Murad received the highest international honor obtainable - the Nobel Prize in Physiology or Medicine. Since 1901, the Nobel Prize in foreign circles has been universally acknowledged as the highest honor. The Nobel Prize was created by a famous Swedish chemist and inventor of dynamite, Alfred Bernhard Nobel, as part of his legacy. The Nobel Prize also includes a gold medal, certificate and prize check. As part of his will, Nobel pledged a large part of his fortune (US\$ 9.2 million) to a fund, which he divided to support 5 separate awards; Physics, Chemistry, Biology, Medicine, Literature and Peace (the Prize in Economics was later added). These prizes would then be awarded in each of the abovementioned fields to academics throughout the world who have made significant contributions to society.

Two years after Dr Murad received the Lasker award; in 1998 he was finally awarded the highest honor - the Nobel Prize in Physiology or Medicine.

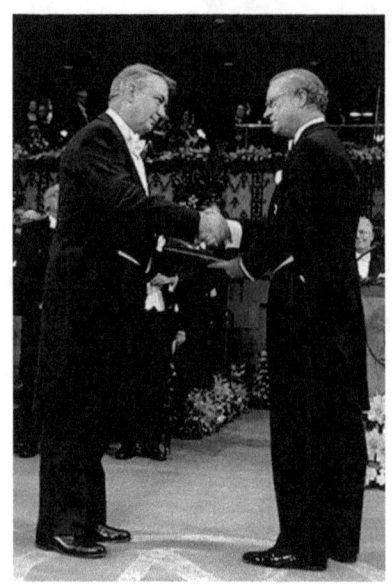

Dr. Murad being awarded the Nobel Prize in 1998 by the Swedish King Carl Gustaf XVI.

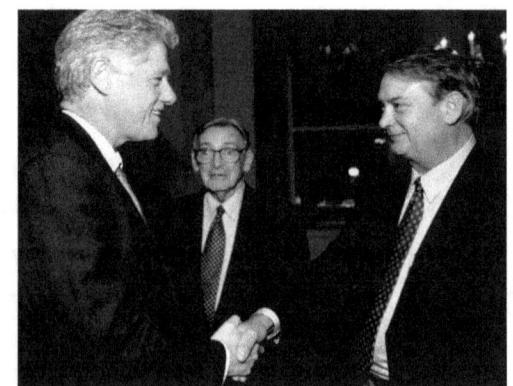

Dr. Murad with former U.S. President Bill Clinton

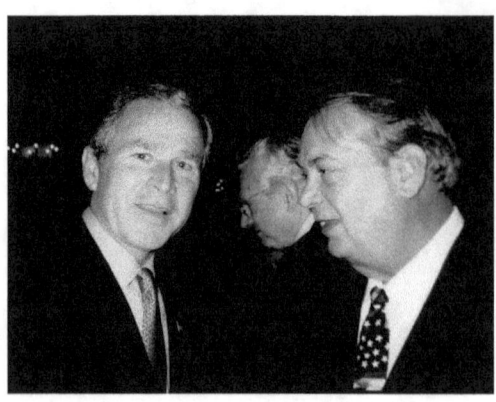

Dr. Murad with former U.S. President George W. Bush

The key to success is by no means sheer luck or chance. From an early age Dr. Murad's aspirations and pursuit of success set him apart from his peers. At the young age of 10, one of Dr. Murad's teachers once asked him what kind of career he might like to pursue later on in life. He replied with clear conviction that he wished to become a doctor, a pharmacologist, a scientist or a teacher. It was in 1960, during his time at university, when Dr. Murad, aged 25, first aspired to winning the Nobel Prize. From this point on, Dr. Murad worked hard to realize this goal. Ten years later in 1970 and at the age of 35, Dr. Murad and his good friend and fellow student Dr. Alfred Gilman speculated on how to achieve their ultimate objective of winning the Nobel Prize. Finally in 1998 at the age of 63, Dr. Murad achieved his lifelong goal of winning the most acclaimed award in the scientific world, the Nobel Prize in Physiology or Medicine. Four years earlier in 1994, Dr. Murad's friend Dr. Alfred Gilman also won the Nobel Prize in Physiology or Medicine for his discovery of G-proteins. Both Dr. Murad and Dr. Gilman are now prominent role models within the scientific world.

Today, even at the grand age of 77, Dr. Murad continues to direct a world-class research team and has no plans to retire from scientific research; "Science is always exciting and I'm still very turned-on." He regularly works 70 hour weeks, and focuses much of his work on research into gliomablastoma, which is one of the most difficult cancers to treat, as well as on enteritis, a disease which claims the lives of millions of Africans each year. Dr. Murad travels frequently, and aims to help promote human health through his international lectures and seminars. He flies over 200,000 km each year to participate in these international visits.

Dr. Murad mentioned in his autobiography that when he was young, he studied hard so that he would have the opportunity to lead an easier life than that of his parents. Yet it is certain that he leads a more hectic life now than his parents ever did. Dr. Murad was once asked if he had ever thought of retirement and a change of lifestyle. "No, I really like the work I am doing now", said Dr. Murad decidedly, "I like to work and have a lot of fun solving problems."

Dr. Murad elected as foreign member of the Chinese Academy of Sciences in landslide vote.

In 2007, Dr. Murad was elected as a foreign member of the Chinese Academy of Sciences, and became the centerpiece of a widely told story in the history of the Chinese Academy of Sciences. The election process for foreign members of the Chinese Academy of Sciences is very strict, and the election happens once every two years. For foreign member candidates, they must obtain at least five academy nominations, each co-opted fellow may nominate up to two candidates. The official shortlist of candidates for election as foreign members is chosen by the official committee of the Chinese Academy of Sciences through discussion and an anonymous ballot. The General Committee of the Chinese Academy of Sciences will then hold an anonymous vote for the final election of foreign members. At least 2/3 of the members who vote in the election, must agree for the election to be effective. Dr. Murad is also a member of various academies of sciences in many other countries, including the United States.

Dr. Murad is a good friend of the Chinese people, and has always been pro-active in collaborating with influential figures of the Chinese scientific world; helping to promote scientific developments and education within China. Since 1999 Dr. Murad has visited China over 30 times, and set foot in over a dozen provinces. He has trained many foreign Chinese nationals, who have worked alongside him in his laboratory. Many of these Chinese have returned home to China to become outstanding and prominent scientists. Since 2000 he has been appointed Honorary Professor at various Chinese universities including Suzhou University, Shanghai Second Medical University, Shanghai University of Traditional Chinese Medicine, Qingdao

University, Beijing Union Medical College (Medical) University, Jiangnan University, and Huazhong University of Science and Technology University. Dr. Murad also acts as scientific advisor, advising on Chinese science and technology strategy, and providing consultation services for many university teams and Chinese state institutions. He is scientific advisor for Shenzhen, a member of the State Biotechnology Institution and Scientific Steering Committee, and a member of the Beijing Institute of Life Sciences Committee. He has played an important consulting role for various cities including Beijing, Shanghai, Hong Kong, Shenzhen, Shijiazhuang and Dalian. He is very willing and eager to help China's higher institutions to develop international relationships and enhance the level of scientific research. Dr. Murad has also collaborated with the Shanghai University of Traditional Chinese Medicine to establish the "Murad Research Institute of Modern Chinese Medicine", and the Shijiazhuang City Government, to develop a large-scale Science and Technology Park – "Murad Science Park".

Dr. Murad's vision for the future of Traditional Chinese Medicine.

As we all know, currently in Europe and N. America, the rate of acceptance for Traditional Chinese Medicine is about 1%, and most people are not particularly interested in Traditional Chinese Medicine. Dr. Murad is a firm supporter of Traditional Chinese Medicine, and plays an active role in helping to promote TCMs throughout the international academic world. Dr. Murad has over 20 years of experience in researching TCMs. In the 1980s, during his time as Director for medical research at Abbott Laboratories, a colleague's wife developed breast cancer and was treated in Hong Kong through a course of Traditional Chinese Medicine. From 1988 to 1990, he visited and gave lectures at the Chinese University of Hong Kong for three consecutive years, and personally witnessed the unique effects of TCMs. It was from that moment on that he developed a strong desire to understand how TCM's worked, and to promote the development of TCMs. Today, Dr. Murad has established the "Murad Research Institute of Modern Chinese Medicine", which focuses on new research into TCMs. He once declared that: "one day in the future, if we are able to determine how TCM's work and successfully identify their active ingredients, the development of Traditional Chinese Medicine will benefit people throughout the world, and not just in China."

The father of nitric oxide and his famous molecule come to China.

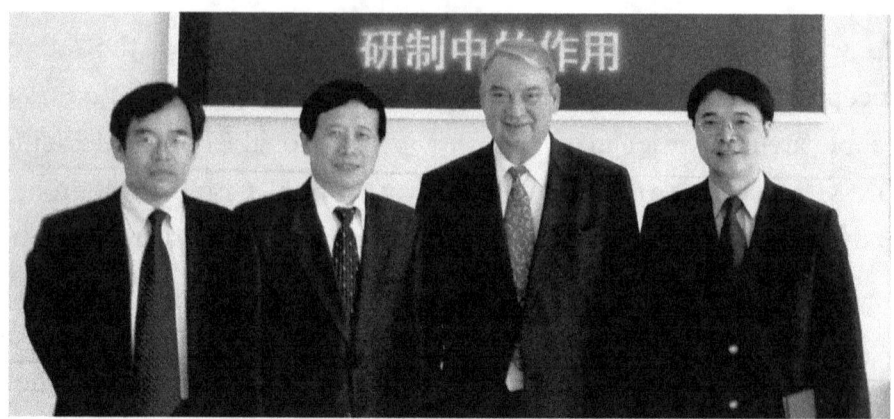

Dr. Ferid Murad (second from right), Dr. Daniel Chen (first from right), and Liu Depei (second from left), member of the Chinese Academy of Engineering and president of Peking Union Medical College.

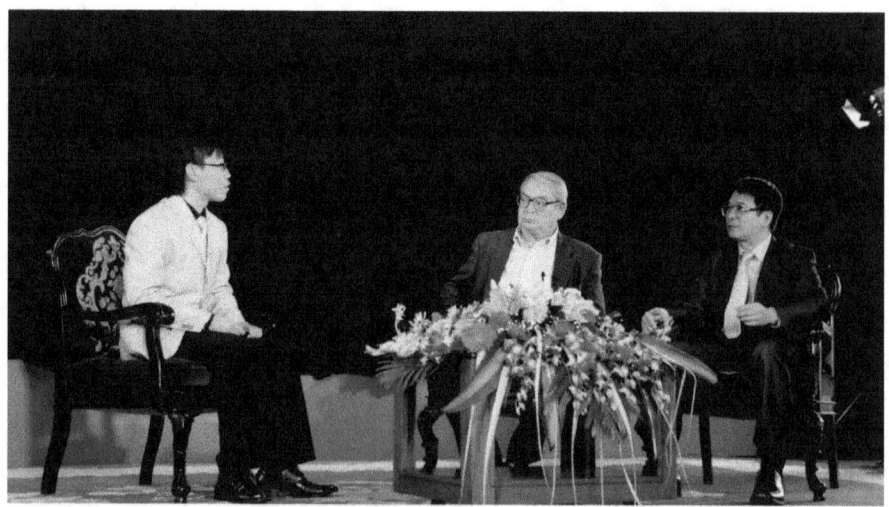

Authors of this book, Dr. Ferid Murad (second from right), and Dr. Daniel Chen (first from right), being interviewed by a CCTV journalist.

Brief Bibliography of Dr. Daniel Chen

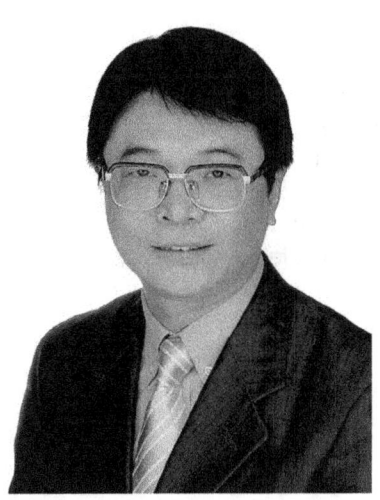

Daniel Chen M.D. Ph.D.

- Senior Adviser of the World Health Organization Southern European Collaboration Centre
- Staff Officer of the United Nations Educational Scientific and Cultural Organization in Paris, France
- PhD Johns Hopkins University
- Medical Doctor MD, PhD

Dr. Daniel Chen, MD, PhD at Johns Hopkins University, a well-known pediatrician, Senior Advisor of World Health Organization southern European collaboration centers, the United Nations Educational Scientific and Cultural Organization Staff Officer of Paris, France has been committed to the promotion and research in nitric oxide for an extended period of time. As student and working partner of 1998 Nobel Prize in Physiology or Medicine laureate Dr. Ferid Murad, Dr. Chen is the sixth generation academic descendant in the field of of cellular signaling science. Dr. Chen won the appreciation and trust of Dr. Murad, and established long term collaboration relationships with many Nobel laureates. Though the encouragement of these great mentors, Dr. Daniel Chen determined to industrialize nitric oxide technology, inheriting the motto and practice of Dr. Murad in saving more people's lives from diseases, and bringing health to mankind in the world.

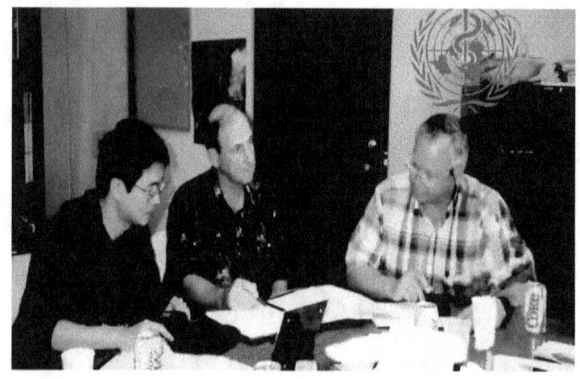

Photograph of Dr. Chen in the meeting of World Health Organization Southern European Collaboration Centre

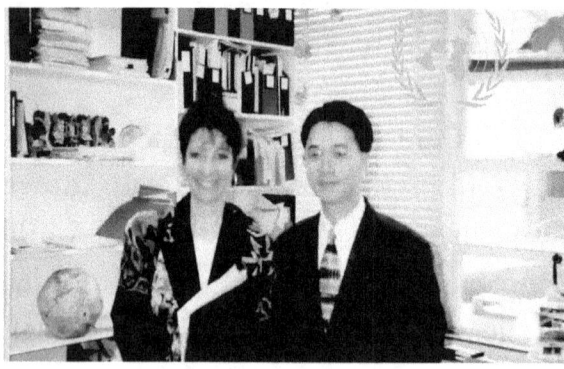

Photograph of Dr. Chen at the office of the United Nations Educational Scientific and Cultural Organization in Paris, France

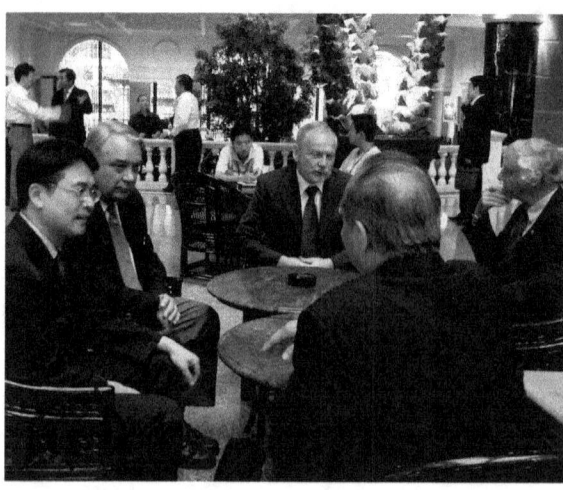

Photograph of Dr. Daniel Chen (1st from left)with Dr. Ferid Murad, 1998 Nobel Prize laureate in Medicine or Physiology; Dr. Hartmut Michel (3rd from right), 1998 Nobel Prize laureate in Chemistry; , Dr. Tsung Dao Lee (2nd from right) 1957 Nobel Prize Physics laureate, the Einstein Science Award winner; and 1998 Nobel Prize chemistry laureate Dr. Robert Huber (1st from right).

Set goal to devote in medicine at a young age, persistence led to success.

Dr. Daniel Chen was born in 1965 into a family with a medical heritage. From the family influence, he set a goal to develop a career in the medical research field at young age. He hoped to help mankind to escape the physical suffering diseases bring medical technology and research.

Dr. Chen obtained bachelor of medical science degree in the year 1991 in Taipei medical school. In 1994, he obtained a master's degree in medical science from Kaohsiung medical school. During the course of these academic years, he passed the medical doctor's certification examinations for Taiwan, USA and China with unwavering devotion. He also passed the qualification exam for senior civil servant rank in the Taiwan government. Such outstanding achievement for a young person in his late twenties exemplified extraordinary wisdom and achievement that very few possess.

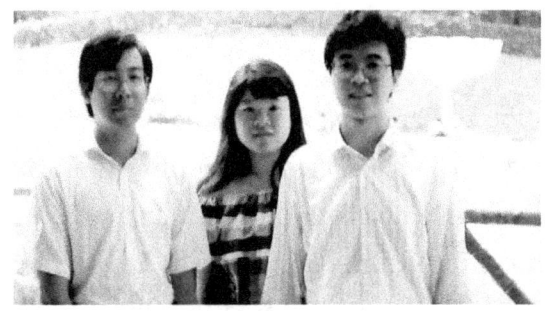

Photograph of Dr. Daniel Chen and his Taipei Medical University fellows

With a deep dedication to the field of medicine, Dr. Chen continued his pursuit and study. In 1997, he obtained the master's degree in public health from the world renowned medical institute- Johns Hopkins University, where in 2000, he obtained the Doctorate of Philosophy in Medicine. This strong foundation serves as a stepping stone for Dr. Chen's future medical research works.

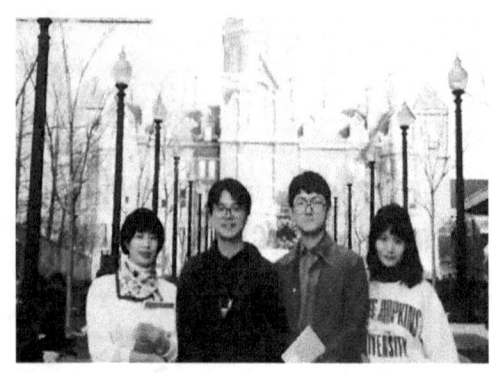

Photograph of Dr. Daniel Chen and his Johns Hopkins University colleagues

Inheriting the mission of "cellular signaling science" from the Nobel Prize laureate

During the time he was obtaining his doctorate degree at Johns Hopkins University, Dr. Daniel Chen met one of the most important persons in his life: the Nobel Prize laureate Dr. Ferid Murad, winner of 1998 Nobel Prize in Physiology or Medicine. Under Dr. Murad's mentorship, Dr. Chen started research in the field of nitric oxide, and entered into the field of cell signaling research. It opened the door for Dr. Chen to industrialize Dr. Murad's Nobel Prize winning nitric oxide technology.

Dr. Murad devoted his life in the research of nitric oxide technology, where he discovered that nitric oxide is an important signaling molecule inside human body. For this discovery, he was awarded the Nobel Prize. Under the mentorship of Dr. Ferid Murad, Dr. Daniel Chen started his research in nitric oxide, and entered the field of cell signaling science.

Up to now, cell signaling research has been though more than a hundred years of development, and the Nobel Prize has been awarded for each period's main discoveries thoughout the generations of scientists in the field of cell signaling. Here is a list of the cell signaling winners' heritage: First generation, 1904, Dr. Ivan Pavlov

XVIII

received the Nobel Prize in Physiology or Medicine; second generation, 1923, Dr. Johns Macleod received the Nobel Prize in Physiology or Medicine; third generation,1947, Dr. Carl Corti and Dr. Gerty Cori husband and wife received the Nobel Prize in Physiology or Medicine; fourth generation, 1971 Dr. Earl Sutherland received the Nobel Prize in Physiology or Medicine; fifth generation, 1994 Dr. Alfred Gilman received The Nobel Prize in Physiology or Medicine; Dr. Ferid Murad is the sixth generation Nobel Prize winner in the history and heritage of cell signaling. This lineage and discovery in cell signaling alongside with the Nobel Prize winners was a greatly talked about story within the field of biology and medicine.

And now, cell signaling science is passed on to the sixth generation, Dr. Murad's student Dr. Daniel Chen, is committed to promoting the most important application- nitric oxide technology in cell signaling science. He hopes to benefit mankind with the nitric oxide technology and ease away the suffering brought by diseases. Dr. Chen is starting a glorious chapter in the heritage of cell signaling history.

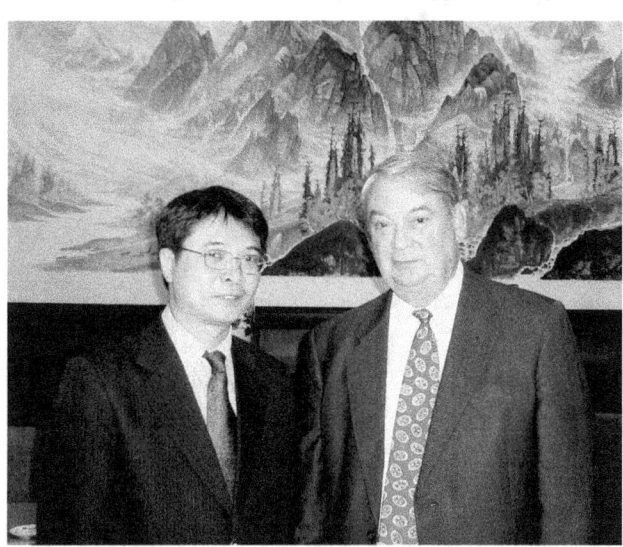

Photograph of Dr. Daniel Chen with winner of 1998 Nobel Prize in Physiology or Medicine, Dr. Ferid Murad

Committed in promoting Nitric Oxide Technology

Nitric oxide has been recognized by the science community as the "Star molecule" since early in the twentieth century. The discovery of nitric oxide and its applications has significant value on the well-being of mankind. Nitric oxide is a prominent molecule in the human body, and it has been widely used in various fields such as medicine, health care, and etc.

Scientists around the globe have been passionately devoted to the research of nitric oxide technology, and this phenomenon caused the nitric oxide related research topic to be the second most published research topic in academic fields. Viagra, the popular drug that's based on nitric oxide technology, has been one of the most important drugs in the world, exemplifying the importance of nitric oxide in the field of medicine. Despite of the fervor that it brings to the field of science and medicine, there are still many people around the world that do not understand the significance of nitric oxide to the health of human body.

Being in the sixth generation of cell signaling science, Dr. Chen has been dedicated to nitric oxide research for more than 20 years. According to Dr. Daniel Chen, 99.9% of the human disease is related to a deficiency in nitric oxide, wherever blood exists, there is nitric oxide. Nitric oxide is essential in the blood circulation system. Once the circulation is hindered, health problems will come flooding. Good nitric oxide regulation in the body is crucial to one's health, and an optimal nitric oxide level in the body is essential to disease prevention and health promotion.

Nitric oxide is especially important in cardiovascular disease prevention and treatment. In the western world, nitric oxide is widely used for cardiovascular related disease treatment. Nitric oxide also plays an important role in the central nervous system, immune system, urinary and reproductive system and various other systems. Ample supply in the body is the key to maintaining optimum health conditions.

Even with this level of importance, nitric oxide is still not well researched in Asian areas; there are very few scientists focusing on the area of nitric oxide.

XX

Industrializing Nitric Oxide technology for the goal of benefiting mankind as a whole

Bearing the selfless ideal of saving lives as a physician, Dr. Daniel Chen is determined to promote nitric oxide technology throughout the world. Together with Dr. Murad, Dr. Chen is also dedicated to new drug development relating to nitric oxide and phosphodiesterase. Many patents were obtained from their nitric oxide technology, in countries such as Taiwan, China, USA and Europe. Industrializing the technology of nitric oxide is a deed that will bring welfare to the multitude.

Dr. Chen said, in order for mankind to benefit from cutting edge biotechnology, we must rely on the industrialization of such technologies. However, there are very few of the existing Nobel Prize technologies that can be industrialized. Biotechnology is a rapidly developing field, and there is urgency to transform it to the commercial realm, via brilliant operational techniques. After decades of research, nitric oxide technology has gradually matured to a level at which it can be industrialized.

To date, nitric oxide technology has been successfully applied to fields such as food, dietary supplements, medicine, skincare products, hair growth products, medical devices and so on. It is to the benefit of mankind's health to have such phenomenal technology industrialized.

Building a sustainable business, and working toward the goal of being among the world's top 500 corporations

The task of promoting nitric oxide technology and products to the entire world cannot be done by oneself; this requires the ability of an international corporate group to take charge in fund raising, consistent new technology development, and integrating all fields of R&D, sales, distribution and manufacturing. Dr. Daniel Chen hopes to continuously develop upon the latest technology, to produce products with the best quality, and distributing them the best channels. This will allow more people to benefit from nitric oxide technology. Bearing such a great ideal in mind, the student of Dr. Murad, Dr. Daniel Chen determined to carry on Dr. Murad's glorious mission of benefiting mankind.

People from the biotechnology field have been moving from the laboratory to the industry, and standing at the frontier of commercialization. The success of such businesses is crucially determined on skillful business operation and management.

Robert Luciano, the CEO of the Global multinational pharmaceutical company -Schering Plough once said a thought pondering sentence: "Pure scientific research is not our goal, we focus creating business opportunities though research; science and business are two sides of a coin; this type of relation enables us to communicate between science, commerce, discovery and application."

As a professional pediatric doctor, Dr. Daniel Chen is prudent and tends to keep a low profile. However Dr. Chen possesses a keen sense and outstanding ability in business operation, management and decision making.

During his service as the general manager of Omnihealth Group Inc., the company's WebMD site, "24drs.com" has been authorized access to the world's largest medical entry website ,WebMD, in the greater China area.

The online joint procurement center of the company has broken the record of the largest online trading in Taiwan in a single transaction- an order of eleven million USD of medical equipment was purchased, and this record brought shock to the medical industry.

During an entrepreneur interview, the reporter asked:"The person who is familiar with the technology field does not necessary have the ability to run a company, while the person with management skills does not necessarily know scientific research. How do you overcome the conflict between scientific research and the industry and establish a connection between them?"

Dr. Daniel Chen replies:"The biotechnology industry requires a management skill backed up by solid scientific knowledge, the leader of biotechnology industry lives in an environment with rapidly evolving market, advancing technology, and constantly changing policies. As a revolutionary leader and manager of biotechnology industry, one has to be constantly updated in new technology and get a good understanding of the trends. One also has to clearly understand the effect that the new technologies bring to the traditional economic and business models, in order to get a hold on this constantly changing industry."

Running a corporation is to simplify the complicated, and while conducting scientific research is to turn a simple idea into a complicated study. As a biomedical company operator, the most important task is to break free from such conflicts.

With medical backgrounds, management and marketing skills, education and training abilities all together, Dr. Daniel Chen has taken the great responsibility of promoting nitric oxide technology and carrying the health of mankind as his own destiny. To fulfill this sacred destiny, he participated in the founding of many biotechnology companies in the United States, Canada, China and Taiwan.

During the growing phase of a corporation, it will face countless difficulties and setbacks. It's like the struggles a sapling needs to go through, to overcome all the environmental interferences and grow into a tree. Through the unique managing skills and the talent in running businesses, Dr. Chen was able to make a breakthrough for his corporations.

Dr. Daniel Chen is a true believer of the saying: "Successful people look for solutions but not excuses." Up to date, as nitric oxide technology becomes the trend of regimen and health care, Dr Daniel Chen is standing strong as the pioneer of this new trend, incorporating the R&D department, manufacturing facilities and distribution systems into a biotechnology empire.

In the future, Dr. Chen is going to follow his teacher Dr. Murad's footsteps, and delve into advancing the research and development of nitric oxide technology, improving the quality of the products, and working toward the goal of being among the world's top 500 corporations, so more people will benefit from nitric oxide and the healthy life that it brings.

Preface

This book was an idea that the authors discussed for several years. We wanted to produce a book that showed the relationship between nutritional supplements and diet to a very important messenger molecule in our body, Nitric Oxide. For my work with Nitric Oxide over the past 35 to 40 years, I received the Nobel Prize in Physiology or Medicine in 1998. We wanted to summarize the importance of Nitric Oxide in a soft, understandable scientific way that the nonscientist would understand. We believe that having some understanding of the biology of Nitric Oxide and relationship with nutritional supplements and diet will promote the readers to take a more proactive role in their health and hopefully in the prevention of some medical diseases.

The authors   Ferid Murad

                            Daniel Chen

Dedication

Dr. Ferid Murad and Daniel Chen want to dedicate this book to their families who have been so supportive over the years and so patient and tolerant regarding their busy work schedules.

Acknowledgement

There are many we wish to acknowledge for their assistance in preparing this book. It is particular important to have excellent assistance when a book is published in many languages (English, Mandarin, Spanish, French and Korean). The assistance of Catherine Fenelon is certainly appreciated as the first two revisions were in English and Mandarin and as a bilingual speaker, she was of great assistance to the authors.

Understanding Nitric Oxide Can Help You Achieve a Healthy Lifestyle

Nitric oxide is one of the simplest yet most fascinating molecules known to man. Interest in the study of nitric oxide reached a new level during the 1990s, but continues to intrigue scientists throughout the world today. In 1992 the Journal Science named nitric oxide "Molecule of the Year", and in 1998, I and two other scientists, Furchgott and Ignarro received the Nobel Prize in Medicine or Physiology for our discoveries concerning nitric oxide as a signaling molecule in the cardiovascular system. My findings demonstrated how nitroglycerine and related drugs work by releasing nitric oxide into the body. Nitric oxide is an important signaling molecule, which controls blood pressure, and regulates blood flow to tissues with a supply of oxygen and nutrition. In fact there are very few tissues in the body that don't have an interaction with nitric oxide.

Since the 1970s there have been over 100, 000 published research papers on nitric oxide. The Nitric Oxide Society and Nitric Oxide Forum are among a wide array of academic circles continuing to promote the importance of research on nitric oxide. In fact growing research suggests that nitric oxide can play a pivotal role in the fight against cardiovascular related deaths, and perhaps many other chronic and fatal diseases. Nitric oxide's key biological functions include its effect on the cardiovascular and immune systems, as well as the circulatory system, central nervous system, and urinary and reproductive systems.

As Director of a world-class research team, member of the U.S. National Academy of Sciences since 1997, and foreign member of the Chinese Academy of Sciences since 2007, I am committed to the research and development of new drugs and nitric oxide based health solutions for improving cardiovascular health and other related diseases. My main objective is to help others to take a more proactive role in their health, through my pioneering research and wealth of knowledge on nitric oxide. Our research and technology is vital to the development of medicines, health supplements, and many other applications.

As a long-standing colleague and good friend of mine, Dr. Daniel Chen has devoted a large part of his career to the promotion of nitric oxide as a unique health solution to many chronic health conditions and diseases. After years of continuously responding to the same questions posed by colleagues and associates concerning nitric oxide and its biological function, Dr. Chen and I decided to publish a book which focuses exclusively on the importance of nitric oxide in human health. It gives me great pleasure to finish this book with him. As a co-author of this book, I'm glad to introduce it to all of you. Our work is an intriguing and illuminating account of the extraordinary properties of nitric oxide, written in an accessible and straight-forward style. This book is a culmination of over 40 years of pioneering research on nitric oxide, and I believe that it will not only benefit readers worldwide, but also serve as an enduring reference and guide for improved well-being and overall health for years to come.

Ferid Murad MD, PhD,
Nobel Laureate 1998
in Medicine.

CONTENTS

PART ONE
NITRIC OXIDE, A HEALTH MESSENGER / 001

For many years, the public perception of Nitric Oxide was primarily negative, owing to the substance's reputation as an atmospheric pollutant released from car exhausts and refuse combustion. It wasn't until the1980s that Ferid Murad, Robert. F. Furchgott and several other scientists were successful in determining the various health benefits of Nitric Oxide– And most importantly their discovery of the function of Nitric Oxide in the vascular system. It was this ground-breaking discovery which was to throw new light on Nitric Oxide as an important "Health messenger"; a discovery for which both Scientists received the Nobel Prize. The importance of Nitric Oxide in treating cardiovascular disease should by no means be underestimated, and new milestones in Nitric Oxide research are being crossed each day.

CONTENTS

We depend on the circulatory system not only to transport oxygen and life-giving substances to the various parts of our body, but also to discharge waste and refuse, constantly supplementing and purifying our bodies in a complete metabolic cycle. There is no doubt that blood and blood vessels are the keystones of human life and health. One might therefore ask: how can we ensure the health of this life giving system? What effect will vascular aging cause to health? What substances or processes are fundamental to the health of this system? Let us explore the processes on which we all depend to find the answers to these universally important questions.

Although state of mind, unlike the physical body, cannot be seen nor touched, it directly influences the amount of enzyme and activity of NOS in the body. Patients' psychological status influences their quality of life, and may also have a significant impact on their physical status, including cardiovascular health. The psychological status

CONTENTS

such as calmness of the mind raises nitric oxide levels in the human body, whilst anger and fear reduce nitric oxide levels. It is important to maintain a good psychological state to keep nitric oxide levels high; for longevity and enhanced quality of life.

CONTENTS

PART FOUR
"3A & 1S" HEALTHCARE METHODS TO LET YOU LIVE ANOTHER 30 YEARS / 130

Nitric oxide can be acquired in such ways as food, moderate exercise and supplements of functional food, while appropriate supplements of antioxidants is another important method to keep nitric oxide formation increased. Therefore, the health-keeping method of "three acquisitions and one supplement" ensures adequate supply of nitric oxide for the body as well as avoids nitric oxide being removed due to rapid oxidation so that the body is always in a healthy state.

CONTENTS

PART FIVE
GROUPS IN NEED OF NITRIC OXIDE / 201

As a kind of nutritional supplement, nitric oxide is involved in the circulation and metabolism of different systems in the human body and shows an extremely important effect for health. What kinds of people need to supplement nitric oxide? As studies show, those in need to supplement include: elderly, mental workers, post-menopausal women, smokers as a group, alcohol drinkers as a group, obese subjects as a group, and hypothyroid persons. Obviously, these are large groups.

PART ONE
NITRIC OXIDE, A HEALTH MESSENGER

The chemical formula for Nitric oxide is NO. NO is a colorless and odorless gas, with a density of 1.3402 kg/m3 and a melting point of -163.6°C. Nitric oxide is water soluble, and can also dissolve in alcohol and sulfuric acid. When exposed to oxygen, NO is easily converted into the highly-corrosive gas, nitrogen dioxide. Under normal conditions nitric oxide is an odorless and colorless gas; while it appears blue in its solid and liquid states.

For many years, the public perception of Nitric oxide was primarily negative, owing to the substance's reputation as an atmospheric pollutant released from car exhausts and refuse combustion. It wasn't until the 1980s when Ferid Murad, Robert. F. Furchgott and several other scientists were successful in determining the various health benefits of Nitric Oxide – And most importantly their discovery of the function of Nitric Oxide in the vascular system. It was this ground-breaking discovery which was to throw new light on Nitric Oxide as an important "Health messenger"; a discovery for which both Scientists received the Nobel Prize. The importance of Nitric Oxide in treating cardiovascular disease should by no means be underestimated, and new milestones in Nitric Oxide research are being crossed each day.

Chapter One
The Cinderella Years of the Miracle Molecule

After enduring negative public perception for many years, in 1992, this ozonosphere damaging, acid rain causing pollutant nitric oxide was honored by *Science* Magazine with the prestigious award, "Molecule of the Year".

In modern society, the exploitation and refining of petroleum and the production of chemical materials is unavoidable. Almost every aspect of our daily lives, be it the products we purchase and use, or the activities that we participate in are inextricably linked to the production of petroleum or products such as gasoline, diesel, kerosene, lubricant, bitumen, plastic and fiber, all of which are refined from petroleum. Gasoline is the most common type of oil product, and is the basis of the vast global automobile industry. It is also responsible for the pollution emitted as part of automobile exhaust, one of the most important pollutions. Atmospheric pollution hazards include severe impact on human health, causing cancer, respiratory diseases and other illnesses. Serious air pollution can also cause large-scale and sudden harm to human body, such as in London and Los Angeles where photochemical smog events cause similar illnesses in thousands of people. One of the substances pollutants emitted as a result of internal combustion in vehicles is nitric oxide.

Nitric oxide in nature is man-made, and as it spreads through the air, it invariably enters our cardiopulmonary circulation. Artificial nitric oxide can cause many problems. While it has not yet been observed whether nitric oxide is poisonous to humans, it is clear nitric oxide has a great impact on human bodies, especially our respiratory systems. With low solubility in water, it is not easily absorbed by the upper respiratory tract and therefore enters the lower respiratory tract and lung with ease, causing diseases such as bronchitis and edema.

Chapter Two
Discovery of the Health Messenger

Hard Course for Discovery of the Health Messenger

In 1980, a budding scientist completed a novel experiment, and published a thesis based on his results. Though the experiment was not intended to be a major one, it would prove to be a turning point in the history of nitric oxide, and would throw new light on a substance that up until that point was not considered by the scientific community to be especially remarkable.

This American pharmacologist, whose name was Robert F Furchgott, published a thesis in the famous magazine, Nature, demonstrating that the relaxing function of acetylcholine (ACh) depends on one diffusible substance released from the endothelium. Subsequently, it was also discovered that the relaxing function of various substances such as bradykinin (BK) also followed the similar mechanism, referred to as "endothelium-derived relaxing factor".

Along with the American magazine Science, the famous British magazine Nature, published by the Nature Publishing Group (NPG), is regarded as the most authoritative and famous scientific magazine in the world. Since 1869 when it was first published, it has reported and commented on the most important breakthroughs in the scientific and technological fields throughout the world. It aims to "place before the general public the grand results of Scientific Work and Scientific Discovery and to give to the general public early information of all advances made in any branch of Natural knowledge throughout the world". 60,000 copies of Nature are issued weekly worldwide, of which one fourth is allocated to libraries and research institutions.

Furchgott's insights into the relaxing properties of one substance were not unprecedented; as early as in the 1870s, it was known that nitrate is a good therapy for ischemic heart disease, though its functioning mechanism was unknown in those days. In the late 19th century, at the time when Alfred Nobel became famous for his research and preparation of high-performance explosives, it had been a surprise to discover that that nitroglycerin (glyceryl trinitrate,or GTN) used in therapy for ischemic heart disease was in fact the main active component of high- performance explosives.

Since the insights of Furchgott's thesis into the relaxation function of nitric oxide were hardly new, why did they provoke so much attention within the scientific field? The reason was that he had proven the existence of such a substance through his cleverly-designed experiment.

On the surface, Furchgott's research showed no direct association with nitric oxide, and was instead concerned with the functioning mechanism of vasoactive substances such as acetylcholine. In 1953, he published the first thesis on acetylcholine and histamine causing the constriction of isolated rabbit vascular strips, which was contrary to the commonly held view at the time that the intravenous injection of acetylcholine or histamine into intact animals would result in vasodilatation. However, he insisted that his experiment showed a good repeatability and was observed without any error, and in the overview of the "Pharmacology of Vascular Smooth Muscle" published in 1955, he proposed a hypothesis, viewing that just as epinephrine can have two receptors, α and β, vascular smooth muscle (VSM) can also contain both motive and inhibitory cholinergic receptors.

With this insight came the corollary: why can stimulating endothelial cells result in VSM relaxation? This time, it seemed to be simple. Initially, it was thought that the stimulation of vascular endothelium would release a substance that diffused to the smooth muscle and caused it to contract. Furchgott seemed to have been struck by a flash of inspiration. He recalled: "when I just woke up that morning, a beautiful experimental design came suddenly into my mind and I immediately conducted the experiment according to this program." The experimental results compiled into his thesis were published the magazine Nature in 1980, which was titled as "Endothelial cells are a necessary factor for acetylcholine to initiate the relaxation of arterial smooth muscle". It should be noted that this article published in Nature magazine had not yet by then definitely proposed the endothelium- derived relaxing factor, and it was not until 1982 when the thesis regarding the endothelium-depended relaxing effect of bradykinin was published in Proceedings of the National Academy of Sciences of the United States of America (PNAS), that the term "endothelium- derived relaxing factor" (EDRF) was formally proposed.

This thesis drew extensive attention in the academic circles and attracted many science workers, including Professor Louis J. Ignarro of California University at Los Angeles, to engage in research on EDRF. EDRF is a variety of unstable compound that can be deactivated by hemoglobin and superoxide anion radical. In collaboration with Furchgott, Ignarro engaged in extensive research on the pharmacological effects of nitroso compounds conducted a series of experiments on the pharmacological effect and chemical nature of EDRF and discovered that like nitric oxide and many nitroso compounds, EDRF can activate soluble guanylate cyclase (sGC), while nitric oxide dilates blood vessels mainly through cyclic guanosine monophosphate (cGMP).

Discovery by Dr. Murad

In the 1960's, cyclic guanosine monophosphate was discovered, as a naturally produced substance, in urine, while the relevant enzymes include guanylate cyclase (GC) used for the synthesis of cyclic guanosine monophosphate, phosphodiesterase for hydrolyzing cyclic guanosine monophosphate and protein kinase selectively activated by cyclic guanosine monophosphate was discovered shortly thereafter.

In 1970, upon finishing his training at National Institute of Health (NIH), Dr. Murad decided to shift the focus of his research from cyclic adenosine monophosphate (cAMP) to cyclic guanosine monophosphate, with the intention of finding the answers to two two questions: (1) how are hormone ligands combined with their receptors to regulate guanylate cyclase? (2) What is the biological effect of the molecule? Understanding of the coupling of receptors to guanylate cyclase is helpful for using preparations or a drug to enhance or control the effect of hormone in some clinical diseases. At The Medical School of University of Virginia, as early as 1977,

Pharmacologist Dr. Murad, who had previously been engaged in research on the effect of nitroglycerin in dilating vessels, discovered that nitro ester drugs and exogenous nitric oxide can both increase the content of cyclic guanosine monophosphate in many tissues. He even proposed that nitro ester may increase the content of cyclic guanosine monophosphate in cells by forming nitric oxide, thus dilating vessels and controlling platelets. At that point most of the scientific research projects focused on one particular topic – active nitro compounds for which he coined the term "nitrovaso-dilators". As early as the 1970s, Dr. Murad and his Trainees had studied the pharmacological effect of nitroglycerin and other organic nitro- compounds with the effect of vasodilatation and discovered that such compounds could all result in the increase of concentration of cGMP in tissues. Such compounds have one property in common: they are all able to produce nitric oxide through internal metabolism. In 1977, Dr. Murad discovered that nitroglycerin and other substances must be metabolized into nitric oxide before they play a role in increasing cGMP and dilation of blood vessels. He therefore began to suspect that nitric oxide might have a regulatory effect on blood circulation on its own, but in those days, there was inadequate experimental evidence to support his hypothesis.

In his early work, Dr. Murad had discovered that guanylate cyclase activity could be detected in different homogenates (including high-speed centrifugal supernatant and homogenate particles). However, in preparing these two types of tissue extracts, enzymatic activity showed different characteristics, of which the most significant was that the activation of homogenate particles with guanosine triphosphate (GTP) showed cooperative kinetics, while the activity of guanylate cyclase was demonstrably typical of Michaelis kinetics. This discovery indicated that the activity of soluble guanylate cyclase represented two different isoforms of the enzyme. Guanylate cyclase was assumed to have different subtypes, but since the crude extract also contains nucleotidase, phosphatase and phosphodiesterase competing for substrate or product, it is impossible to eliminate non-reliable false data. It took Murad exactly 12 years to purify, demonstrate, clone, express and re-demonstrate the isoforms of the enzyme before this problem was thoroughly resolved.

Through experiments, Dr. Murad discovered that some substances, including sodium azide, nitrite and hydroxylamine, can activate guanylate cyclase. In different tissues, including tracheal smooth muscle, sodium azide, nitrite and hydroxylamine can also increase the level of cyclic guanosine monophosphate. The level of such cyclic guanosine monophosphates increases in association with smooth muscle relaxation, showing a direct relationship. Used as a treatment for clinical angina since the 1770s, nitroglycerin can also activate soluble guanylate cyclase and increase the level of cyclic guanosine monophosphate in different tissues including tracheal gastrointestinal and vascular smooth muscle, resulting in smooth muscle relaxation.

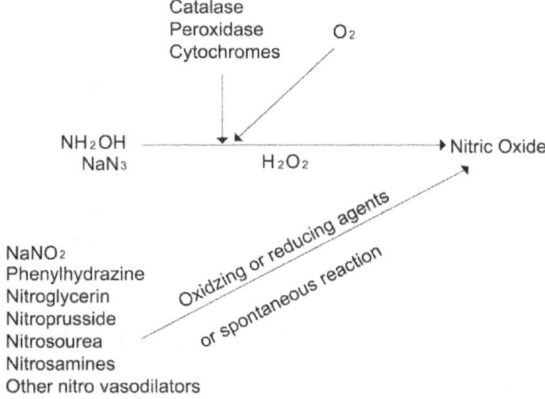

Nitric oxide precursors and "nitrovasodilators" are transformed in the body to nitric oxide (e.g. nitroglycerin, etc. in the body generates and releases nitric oxide).

Dr. Murad placed these relaxants of tracheal, gastrointestinal and vascular smooth muscles in the growing list of soluble guanylate cyclase activators which he called "nitro vasodilatation agents", believing that they could be transformed into nitric oxide. This was because nitric oxide produced chemically in the laboratory was able to activate soluble guanylate cyclase in all the tests. The functioning mechanism of such nitric oxide precursors was determined accordingly.

Dr. Murad hypothesized that nitric oxide could play the role of an intracellular messenger regulating hormone and drug levels: i.e., whereby this free radical is an endogenous messenger molecule. As the activating function of purified soluble guanylate cyclase takes place under a nanomolar concentration of nitric oxide, and the determination method of nitric oxide and its oxidation products, nitrite and nitrate is not sensitive enough, it was seven or eight years after the development of new techniques for analyzing nitric oxide that this hypothesis, which at the time was subject to widespread doubt within the academic community was decisively demonstrated and accepted.

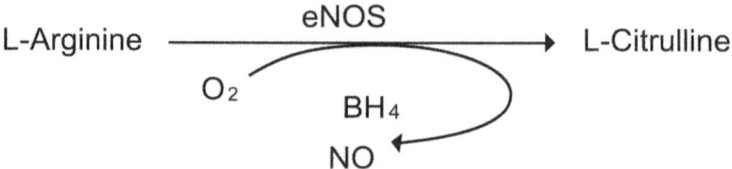

Formation of enzymatically formed nitric oxide (under the effect of endothelial NOS, NOS generates L-citrulline and releases nitric oxide from the amino acid L-arginine)

The research of Dr. Murad not only explored the mechanism of nitric oxide for dilating vessels in the body, but also developed an approach for researching and developing new drugs and cosmetics. The technology by which Dr. Murad conducted his research was a combination of nitrovasodilators and drugs which can produce nitric oxide. The nitrogen reagent is nitrite or extracts of plants rich in nitrite, while the acid reagent is an organic or inorganic acid such as vitamin C and citric acid. To use, first clean the skin, apply an appropriate amount of nitrogen-reagent cosmetics and then apply the acid-reagent cosmetics. The two cosmetics slowly react and release nitric oxide for infiltration into the skin to increase the blood flow in capillaries and promote the formation of collagen, and thus improve skin quality and wound healing.

It should be noted that as early as the late 19th century, German scholar,) Peter Griess studied and published the detection method for nitrite, but at that time its relationship with nitric oxide was not understood. Being the end product of oxidation and metabolism of nitric oxide in water solution, nitrite is relatively stable, and thus the improved Griess method is still, by now, one of the simplest and most common methods for indirectly detecting nitric oxide oxidation products in labs.

An accomplished disciple owes his accomplishment to his great teachers——Passing the flame of Noble Prize

Dr. Turhon Murad most definitely can tell the story of hearing his eldest brother, Ferid Murad, and his friend Al Gilman discussing what it would take to win the Nobel Prize in physiology or medicine during a dinner party back in 1970.

The conversation at the time seemed ridiculous. Not so in hindsight, considering Gilman went on to do that very thing in 1994, as did Ferid four years later for his discovery on how nitric oxide affects the dilation of blood vessels, leading to a host of medical breakthroughs, including Viagra.

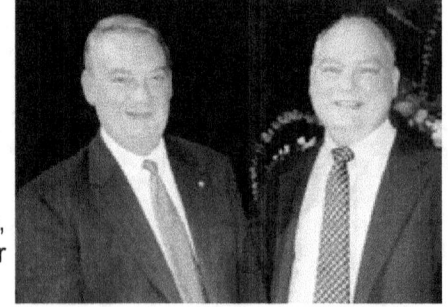

Nobel Prize winner in medicine, Dr. Ferid Murad, with his brother Dr. Turhon Murad, Anthropology.

The research field of cellular communication entered into a new era as nitric oxide was discovered as a cellular messenger.

The cell is the basic structural and functional unit of all known living organisms. And all vital functions of an organism occur within cells. Changes in human genetics, development and physiological function are all closely associated with cells. Cell metabolism forms the basis of all human functions, including substrate metabolism, energy metabolism and information communication. Communication between cells provides the necessary conditions for maintaining growth, development and the division of multi-cell organisms.

Where varying types of cell communication between normal cells is observed; the metabolism and development of organisms are all subject to the regulation and control of information related to genetics and environmental changes; the science of cell communication can be referred to as the organism's sensitivity and response to the external environment; whereas hormones, neurotransmitters and so on help facilitate cell communication.

From the very first macroscopic animals, to organs and cells and present day genetic structures, the cognition level of cell communication science is continually developing and expanding. During this course of evolution, cognitive development has greatly expanded and changed all human understanding, as well as producing a series of Nobel prizes.

Only by understanding how communication is conducted between cells will it be possible to solve the riddle of human life. So how do cells communicate with each other? And how then is information processed following cell communication?

The First Messenger of Cell Communication -- Hormones
Theory of the Conditioned Reflex--Pavlov (Winner of the 1904 Nobel Prize in Physiology and Medicine)

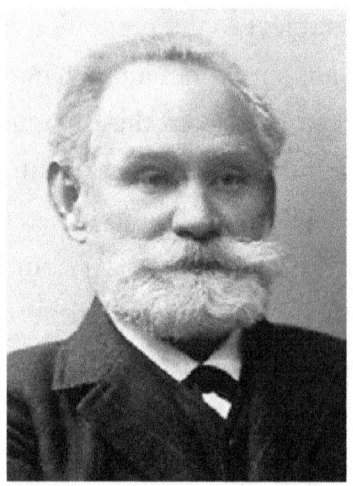

Pavlov, Winner of the 1904 Nobel Prize in Physiology and Medicine

In the late 19th century, whilst researching digestive physiology, Pavlov discovered the main role of the nervous system in the whole digestive process. He also found that the Vagus Nerve, the tenth cranial nerve located in the gastric wall, was associated with gastric secretion. When various sense organs are stimulated by food, the taste organ delivers a message to the brain via the nervous system, whereupon the Vagus nerve allows gastric secretion to occur. It is the theory of conditional reflex. For this, he won the "Nobel Prize" in physiology and medicine and became the first Russian scientist to achieve such an honor. For his outstanding achievement in digestive physiology, Pavlov was honored with the 1904 Nobel Prize in Physiology and Medicine and became the first physiologist worldwide to win the Nobel Prize.

Discovery of Insulin (Hormone) —— Banting and Macleod (Co - winners of the 1923 Nobel Prize in Physiology and Medicine)

Pavlov noticed that after a dog consumed food, the dog's stomach required great efforts to grind the food. With the food entering the small intestine, the pancreas located behind the stomach would then secrete pancreatic juice and immediately deliver it to the small intestine for mixing with the ground food and for digestion. How does the pancreas receive the message from the small intestine? It was also noticed that when hydrochloride is injected into the dog's duodenum, it can cause pancreatic secretion to increase markedly. In his opinion, this phenomenon resulted from nervous reflex. However, in experiments, with the nerve cut off, hydrochloride entering the duodenum can also cause pancreatic secretion to increase. In the opinion of Pavlov, it was due to the reason that the nerve was blocked off.

In 1900, with a brand-new method, the young British physiologist, Starling designed an experiment: scraping duodenal mucosa from one dog and filtering it before injecting it into another dog; consequently, the dog's pancreatic secretion increased markedly. Finally in 1902, after two more years of experiments, together with Bayliss, he proved the existence of secretin. When acid chyme entered the duodenum, intestinal mucosal cells secreted secretin, which was delivered through blood to cause the pancreas to secrete more pancreatic juice. Hence, in the early 20th century, British scientists Bayliss and Starling first discovered secretin from the extracts of small-intestine mucosa and took the lead in proposing the concept of hormones. Through the transportation of fluids in the body, hormones are delivered to the specific functional parts so as to induce a biological effect.

Secretin is a great discovery in the history of endocrinology, which has helped man to discover not only a new chemical substance, but also a new concept and a new field of coordinating organic functions, shaking the idea that the organism was completely regulated by nerves. It indicated that in addition to the nervous system, there was a way of coordinating the activities of remote organs through the delivery of chemical substances: hormonal coordination.

Since 1902 when Bayliss and Starling discovered the first type of hormone, there began a worldwide upsurge for the search of hormones and this set the stage for man to explore such matters as hormones. During the upsurge, the most eye-catching achievement was that in 1920, with the help and support of British physiologist Macleod from the University of Toronto, Canadian physiologist Banting extracted, identified and prepared insulin together with another two assistants.

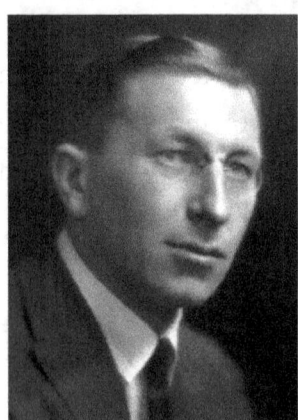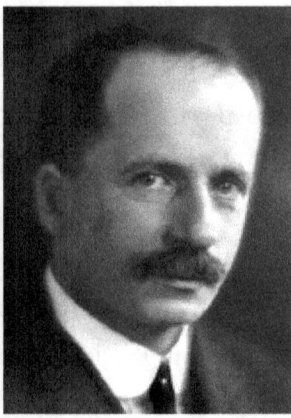

Banting (L) and Macleod (R), Co-winners of the 1923 Nobel Prize in Physiology and Medicine

"For the discovery of insulin", Banting and Macleod were awarded the 1923 Nobel Prize in Physiology and Medicine. In the subsequent five decades, a huge number of hormones were discovered and identified, but such research was mostly concentrated on animals and on organs, yet little research was done on cells.

From hormone to second messenger—Dr. and Mrs. Cori (Co-winners of the 1947 Nobel Prize In Physiology and Medicine and teachers to Dr. Murad's mentor)

Dr. Carl Cori and Mrs. Gerty T. Cori were famous scientists. Both of them were born in Prague (Capital of Czechoslovakia) and both received medical doctorate degrees in 1920. They were married in 1920 and moved to Buffalo, USA for work in 1922. Later on, when they moved to Saint Louis, Mrs. Cori joined in the research work of her husband. They won the Nobel Prize in 1947 when both of them were engaged as professors of biochemistry at Washington University of Medicine, USA. When Dr. and Mrs. Cori came to the USA, their initial research was on the impact of insulin and epinephrine in animals. Their research on glucose metabolism was to extract enzyme tissues separated from integral animal bodies.

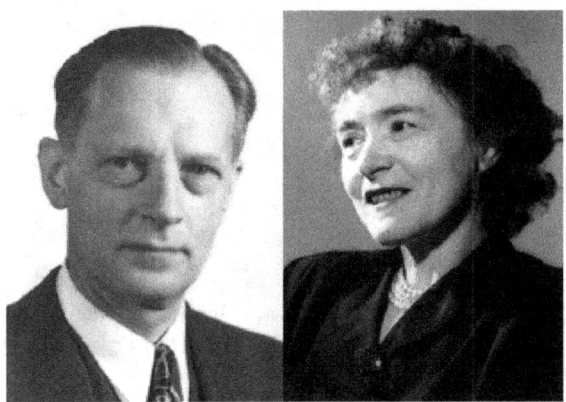

Dr. & Mrs. Cor-Co-winners of the 1947 Nobel Prize in Physiology and Medicine

In the 1930s, Dr. and Mrs. Cori discovered that glycogenolysis was regulated and controlled by hormones. They examined the biological process for the metabolism of glycogen into glucose and showed a clear picture of the enzymes and intermediate metabolites involved. In other words, they discovered the approach for the metabolism of glycogen into glucose, and were able to explain the relation of enzyme reactions between glycogen and glucose and proved how such reactions were controlled by in vivo physiological factors. In 1947, Dr. and Mrs. Cori won the Nobel Prize for their research on glucose metabolism.

In the 1940s, the Cori Laboratory started to study the impact of hormones and discovered that epinephrine and glucagon could promote glycogenolysis, but the particular mechanism was not clear.

Cyclic Adenosine Monophosphate (cAMP) - Dr. Sutherland (winner of the 1971 Nobel Prize in Physiology and Medicine and teacher to Dr. Murad)

In 1947, Sutherland came to the laboratory of Dr. & Mrs. Cori for further research on the enzymatic reaction of glycogen and discovered the rate-limiting enzyme in the process of such glycogenolysis-- phosphorylase is the functional target of epinephrine and glucagon. It was discovered that epinephrine promotes glycogenolysis by regulating the activity of phosphorylase. In cells, phosphorylase was discovered, which could cause phosphorylation of key enzymes for activation in the process of glycogenolysis and also

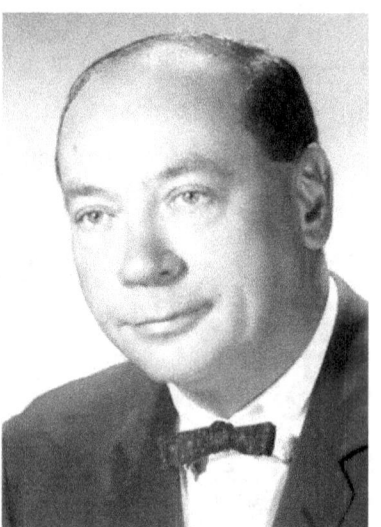

Sutherland, Winner of the 1971 Nobel Prize in Physiology and Medicine

to promote glycogenolysis. Phosphorylase has two forms: active and inactive, the difference between these two is in their phosphate groups: the one with phosphate is active and the one without phosphate is inactive. This result indicated that epinephrine causes the breakdown of glycogen by promoting the phosphorylation reaction of phosphorylase. Epinephrine increased the production of a "heat stable factor" that was cyclic adenosine monophosphate (cAMP). The cyclic AMP increased the activity of phosphorylase and represented the first intracellular messenger to be discovered. For this, Sutherland won the 1971 Nobel Prize.

In this paradigm epinephrine (adrenaline) is the first messenger. Upon entering the cell, information from the first messenger will produce the second messenger cyclic AMP within the cell. In regard to this research topic, the students of Sutherland started the relevant research in the 1960s. Alfred Gilman was a good friend of Murad and was 4 years hehind Murad in the MD- PhD programme. Gilman concentrated his research on the hormonal regulation of the second messenger cAMP, playing a role in epinephrine, and co-discovered GTP (guanosine triphosphate) binding protein with Martin Rodbell.

Nitric Oxide — Dr. Murad (1998 Nobel Prize in Physiology and Medicine)

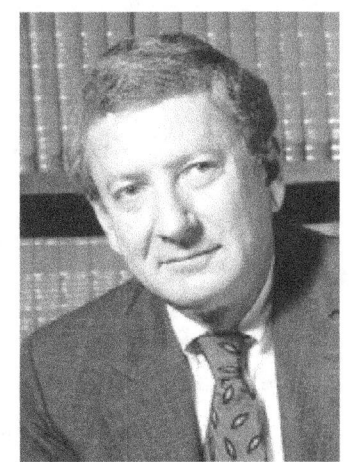

Soon after the discovery of cAMP, Murad joined the laboratory of Sutherland and became aware of the important role of the second messenger in the information delivery system of hormones. He worked as a student with Southerland, and Rall was to prove that epinephrine's effect to increase cyclic AMP synthesis was modulated through the beta adrenergic receptor. He also discovered that another hormone, acetylcholine inhibited

Alfred Gilman, co-Winner of the 1994 Nobel Prize in Physiology and Medicine with Martin Rodell this reaction. Ten years later he switched his research to another cyclic nucleotide, cyclic GMP, believing that it would also be an intracellular messenger. Upon starting the research on a new type of second messenger cGMP (cyclic guanosine monophosphate) for the regulation of enzymes, he discovered how cGMP was generated in cells and its powerful physiological function. As early as the 1870s, it was discovered that organic nitrates showed good therapeutic effects for ischemic heart disease with angina pectoris, or heart pain, but its biological mechanism was not understood in those days. As a pharmacologist, Murad had independently in the 1970's undertaken the research on the vasodilation effect of nitroglycerin at the University of Virginia. As early as in 1977, he discovered that by forming NO, nitrate drugs increased intracellular cGMP for vasodilation. Subsequently, Dr. Murad conducted a series of in-depth research studies. In particular, he discovered how the miraculous properties of the signaling molecule NO promoted the production of cGMP and how it affected the cardiovascular system. Gilman and Murad won the 1994 and 1998

Nobel Prizes respectively.

In 1953, Sutherland became a professor and a chairman of the Medical and Pharmacology Departments at Case Western Reserve University and continued with his research on the function of epinephrine regulating phosphorylase. In 1956, as a young PhD graduate, Theodore Rally went to work in Sutherland's laboratory and delivered a breakthrough in the relevant research.

In 1963, cyclic guanosine monophosphate (cGMP) was discovered, as a product found in urine, while the relevant enzymes including guanylate cyclase (GC) used for the synthesis of cGMP, phosphodiesterase for hydrolyzing cGMP and protein kinase selectively activated by cGMP were discovered in the late 1960s and early 1970s. In 1957, researchers in Sutherland's laboratory discovered the glycogenolysis effect of cAMP as the second messenger to regulate epinephrine and glucagons. Later in the late 1960's and early 1970's he also began some work with cyclic GMP. In those days, people researching cGMP were far fewer than those on cAMP. During his study as a doctoral candidate, Dr. Murad mainly researched the effects of catecholamine on cAMP synthesis and found out whether such effects could be mediated through epinephrine α or β receptors and also discovered that choline esters could inhibit the activity of adenylate cyclase. In 1970, Dr. Murad finished his clinical training and fellowship training and started his career in independent research at the University of Virginia, with his research direction changing gradually from cAMP to cGMP. He found that azide, hydroxylamine and nitrite not only can activate quanylate cyclase in cell-free extracts, but also can increase the cGMP content of many tissues and cells including brain, liver and some cultured cells. Shoji Katsuki, a Japanese doctoral candidate in Murad's laboratory, devised the tracheal smooth muscle (TSM) system from beef lung for detecting the effect of cAMP and cGMP on the smooth muscle. The system proved to be extremely successful and was later applied in different tissues and thus established as an excellent experimental platform.

In different tissues, including tracheal smooth muscle, sodium azide, nitrite and hydroxylamine can increase levels of cGMP. The level of cGMP increase in association with smooth muscle relaxation, showing a straight-line dose response relationship. As a drug applied for clinical angina since the 1870s, nitroglycerin can also activate soluble guanylate cyclase and increase, in different tissues including tracheal smooth muscle, cGMP levels, resulting in smooth muscle relaxation. Another smooth muscle relaxant, sodium nitroprusside (SNP) also has a similar effect. The ever increasing list of soluble guanylate cyclase activators, which are also the relaxants of tracheal, enterogastric and vascular smooth muscles and which he called nitro vasodilation agents or nitrovasodilators, are believed to be transformed into NO. Since such hormones and drugs can increase the formation of the endogenous precursor, he presented the hypothesis that nitric oxide can play a role as an intra-cellular messenger regulating hormones and drugs. As the activating function of purified soluble guanylate cyclase takes place under nano-molar concentrations of nitric oxide, and the determination method of nitric oxide and its oxidation products, nitrite and nitrate are not sensitive, it was seven or eight years before more sensitive analytical techniques of nitric oxide were developed. Thus this hypothesis was widely doubted in academic circles in those days was finally decisively demonstrated and accepted.

Creating an endearing Nobel legacy - Passing the torch

Dr. and Mrs. Cori won the Nobel Prize in 1947 for their research on glycogen metabolism. They discovered the approach for the metabolism of glycogen into glucose and proposed that the conversion between glycogen and glucose was subject to the regulation and control of enzymes.

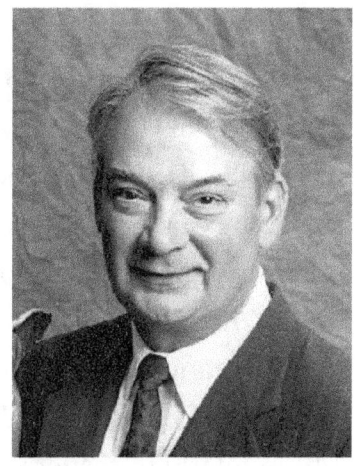

Ferid Murad, Winner of the 1998 Nobel Prize in Physiology and Medicine

As a student of Dr. and Mrs. Cori, Sutherland carried out further research on the enzymatic reaction of glycogen metabolism and discovered that such conversion was subject to the regulation and control of epinephrine and that the hormone increases the formation of cyclic AMP the second messenger in the human body. For this, Sutherland won the Nobel Prize in 1971. Upon entering the cell, the information of the first messenger would create the second messenger. As a student of Sutherland, Gilman concentrated his research on the regulation of the second messenger cAMP, by epinephrine and discovered G-protein. And then as a student of Sutherland, Murad concentrated his research work on a new type of second messenger; cGMP for the regulation of enzymes, and discovered how cGMP was produced in cells and its powerful physiological function. In particular, he discovered how the miraculous properties of the signaling molecule NO promoted the production of cGMP and how it affected the cardiovascular system. Gilman and Murad won the 1994 and 1998 Nobel Prizes respectively. From Dr. and Mrs. Cori to Murad, the torch was passed on for two more generations, spanning five decades, and indicating that it is not haphazard but perhaps inevitable for a line of successful Nobel Prize winners to be intrinsically linked through an academic research network.

As the fourth generation, student of Murad and a doctor from Johns Hopkins University, one of the most famous medical schools worldwide, Dr. Daniel Chen is devoted to the research of nitric oxide technology and its potential applications. In 2010, with the goal of improving medical developments in China and promoting the health of the Chinese people, Dr. Daniel Chen joined hands with Dr. Murad, to bring various applications of NO technology to China, creating a new chapter in academic development. Other Chinese (more than 140 in total) are scattered around the world and conducting reported research.

From Pavlov to Murad, the torch has been passed on for more than a century and the laboratory of Dr. and Mrs. Cori was successful in cultivating six Nobel Prize winners. Obviously, it is not simply by chance that such a line of Nobel Prize winners was created.

Family Tree Diagram of Cell Communication Science

Winner of the 1904 Nobel Prize in Physiology or Medicine—**Pavlov**

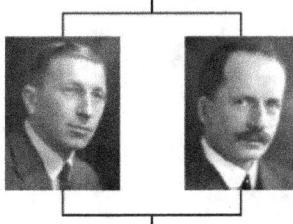

Co-winners of the 1923 Nobel Prize in Physiology or Medicine—**Banting & Macleod**

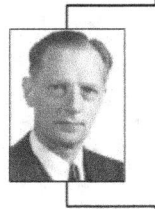 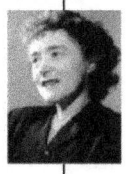

Co-winners of the 1947 Nobel Prize in Physiology or Medicine— **Mr. & Mrs. Cori** (teachers to Dr. Murad's mentor)

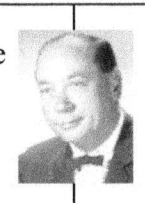

Winner of the 1971 Nobel Prize in Physiology or Medicine— **Dr. Sutherland** (teacher of Dr. Murad)

Winner of the 1998 Nobel Prize in Physiology or Medicine — **Dr. Murad**

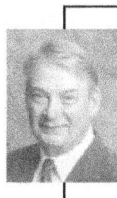

Winner of the 1994 Nobel Prize in Physiology or Medicine — **Dr. Gilman**

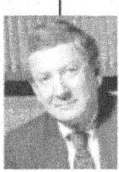

Johns Hopkins University, USA M.D., Ph.D. — **Daniel Chen**

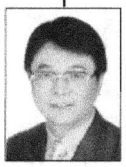

Winning the Nobel Prize

Not long after nitric oxide was awarded "Molecule of the Year, Murad and Furchgott both won the Lasker Medical Award in 1996. The Lasker Award is known informally as "America's Nobel" and 76 winners of the Lasker Awards, primarily in basic medical research have gone on to receive the Nobel Prize.

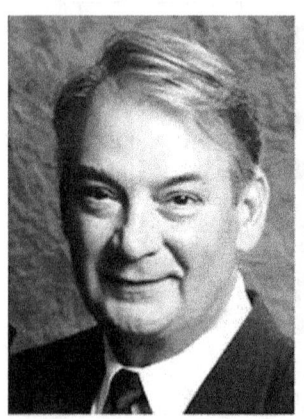 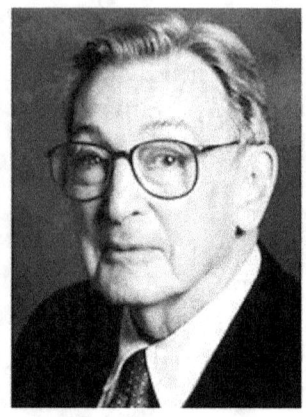 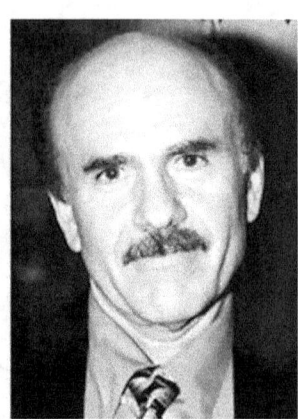

Ferid Murad   Robert F.Furchgott   Louis J.Ignarro

1998 Nobel laureates in Physiology or Medicine: Ferid Murad, Robert F Furchgott, and Louis J Ignarro

scientists, Murad, Furchgott and Ignarro, for their discovery concerning nitric oxide as a signaling molecule in the cardiovascular system .

Upon winning the prize, the Nobel Committee stated: "The Swedish Nobel Prize Committee is pleased to award the prize to the research on the effect of nitric oxide on cardiovascular functions. It is common knowledge that the winners of 1998 Nobel Prize for Physiology or Medicine were: Ferid Murad, Robert F. Furchgott and Louis J. Ignarro, and that Salvad or Moncada missed out on winning the Nobel Prize for Physiology or Medicine, as he was not one of the pioneer discoverers of nitric oxide effects. It is also known that Alfred Nobel had angina pectoris and refused to use nitroglycerin. Had Nobel foreseen their awards, he might have used nitroglycerin to extend his life."

Death of Nobel

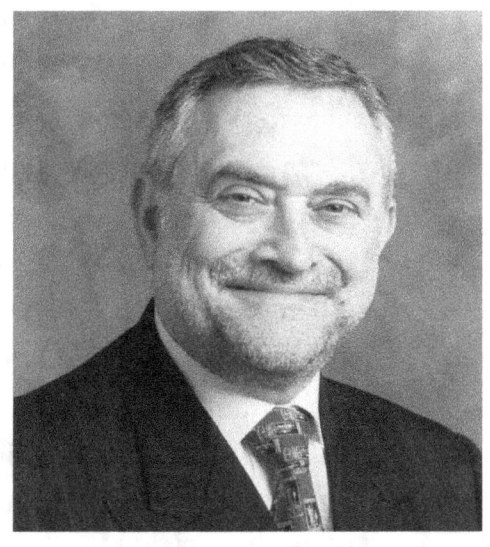

Salvador Moncada, the famous scientist who closely missed out on the 1998 Nobel Prize in Physiology or Medicine.

Alfred Bernhard Nobel (1833.10.21—1896.12.10) was a Swedish chemist, engineer, inventor, manufacturer of military equipment and inventor of explosives. Using his huge fortune, his last act was to found the "Nobel Prize". He was further commemorated in the scientific community in 1957 with the discovery of the 102nd element, nobelium, which also bore his name. In his life, Nobel was responsible for many inventions and creations, making world-famous contributions to science and technology and bringing huge benefits to mankind. Of all, one dramatic invention was associated with nitric oxide. In 1864, Nobel discovered that the extremely evaporative and powerful explosive nitroglycerin, previously synthesized by Italian chemists in 1847, became considerably more stable and less explosive when combined with diatomite. On the basis of this discovery, Nobel successfully developed an explosive that could be detonated without excessive risk to the user. Industrialized production of safe explosives brought Nobel great honor and huge fortune with which he was able to found the top award of science in the world, Nobel Prize. In the late years of his life, Nobel suffered from heart disease and his doctor recommended nitroglycerin to him, but Nobel refused. This was due to his recollection of his days developing nitroglycerin- based explosives, when he discovered that with prolonged exposure nitroglycerin would result in a fierce vascular headache. In 1896, Nobel passed away due to a stroke. Yet if he had listened to the advice of the doctor and used nitroglycerin in time, he might have lived longer and created more fortune for mankind. Nitroglycerin can effectively relieve angina, but its mechanism had puzzled physicians and pharmacologists for more than one hundred years until the 1977 when the American pharmacologist Murad found that it relaxed smooth muscle by forming nitric oxide. Later Furchgott and Ignarro confirmed Murad's discovery that nitroglycerin and other organic nitrates relax vascular smooth muscle by releasing nitric oxide gas and dilating blood vessels.

Health Messenger in the Human Body

Nowadays, it is widely known that nitric oxide plays the role of an important signaling molecule in the human body and small molecules of nitric oxide generated in the human body can pass through any cells to reach any tissue so that the signal is distributed from one part of the human body to other parts, exercising the function of transmitting signals. Nitric oxide helps to control the flow of blood to different parts of the human body for vascular dilation (thereby improving blood flow in vessels), keeps vessels clean and open, maintains a normal blood pressure and effectively reduces the burden of the heart. In addition, nitric oxide is also an effective weapon against germs, viruses, and other infections, and is able to assist in the extermination of various pathogens, and thus protecting human health. Therefore, nitric oxide is a "health messenger" in the human body and an important element for the maintenance of human health.

Vascular EDRF

The production of nitric oxide in the body occurs when arginine is converted to nitric oxide (and citruline) under the effect of NOS. NOS can be basically classified into three types: endothelial (NOS3), neuronal (NOS1) and inducible (NOS2). NOS 1 and 3 are constitutive enzymes, existing under normal physiological conditions; NOS2 is an inducible enzyme, which can be produced through induction under special conditions.

As an EDRF, the main function of nitric oxide generated in the endothelium is to cause vessels to dilate, reduce vascular resistance, lower blood pressure, inhibit platelet adhesion and aggregation, inhibit leukocyte adhesion and migration, reduce smooth muscle growth and prevent atherosclerosis (AS) and thrombus formation.

As a neurotransmitter other than adrenaline, acetylcholine, and other substances, nitric oxide generated in peripheral nerves and the brain plays a very important role in regulating peripheral output nerves such as those in vessels, the cavernosum, the gastrointestinal tract, the urinary tract, the tracheal muscle and the anococcygeal muscle.

Nitric oxide produced through induced nitric oxide (NOS2) regulates inflammation through multiple channels, and plays a very important role in controlling immune response. Nitric oxide has the effect of killing germs, fungi, parasites and tumor cells. Additionally, many of the pathological processes after infections and rheumatoid arthritis, (including shock, tissue damage, cell apoptosis, etc.) are associated with excessive production of nitric oxide and a toxic byproduct peroxynitrite.

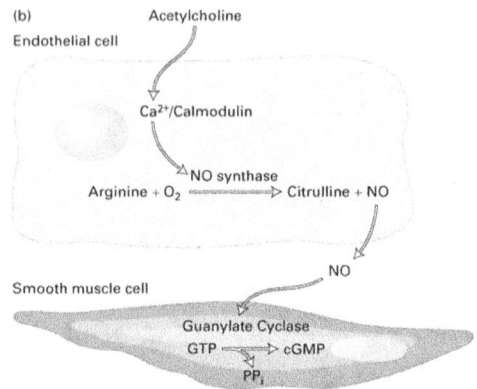

Chapter Three
Physiological Function of Nitric Oxide

At present, modern medical research indicates that the main physiological effects of nitric oxide for the cardio-cerebrovascular system include vasodilatation and the prevention of platelet aggregation, among others. Stimulation by such chemical substances as acetylcholine or bradykinin, in vascular endothelial cells causes the calcium channel on the cell membrane to open, the concentration of calcium in cells increases; and then through calmodulin (CaM), the activation of NOSallows arginine to generate nitric oxide that passes through endothelial cell membranes to diffuse into the surrounding smooth muscle cells, thereby activating guanylate cyclase, generating cGMP, and thus relaxing smooth muscle.

Regulation of vascular tension

Nitric oxide can reduce the response of arteries to noradrenaline stimulation, resulting in decreased vascular tension.

Regulation of myocardial contractility

Many in vivo and in vitro experiments have indicated that nitric oxide has the effect of inhibiting myocardial contractility. In their research, scientists conducted an experiment, where a guinea pig was injected with endotoxin in its peritoneum; 4 hours afterward, the heart was taken out to determine the contractility of a single cell and it was observed that the contractility of myocardial cells had declined.

Such effects can be reversed by a NOS inhibitor N- nitro-L-NAME, preventing lipopolysaccharide (LPS) to activate iNOS for generation of nitric oxide, so as to inhibit myocardial contraction. Additionally, after scientists directly applied nitric oxide and the nitric oxide donor sodium nitroprusside to the in vitro ventricular myocyte of a normal guinea pig, it was also observed that contractility of myocardinal cells decreased, directly proving the inhibiting effect of nitric oxide on myocardinal contractility.

Regulation of endothelial antithrombotic effects

According to some research, nitric oxide is an effective platelet inhibitor. Endothelial injury causes platelet adhesion and aggregation, while nitric oxide can inhibit the platelet response. The antithrombotic effect of an endothelial surface depends, to a great extent, on the synergistic effect of nitric oxide and prostacyclin. It is reported that nitric oxide and prostacyclin show synergistic anti-aggregation effects on platelets, and can reduce or inhibit partial vasospasm and thrombosis.

Regulation of the interaction of neutrophilic granulocyte and endothelial cells and vascular permeability

Nitric oxide can inhibit the effects of various blood elements for aggregation and adhesion to vascular endothelial cells. A NOS inhibitor can promote the adhesion and migration of neutrophilic granulocytes, causing the permeability of micro-vessels to enhance promptly and the leakage of vascular albumin to increase, and thus indicating acute inflammation.

The anti-adhesion effect of nitric oxide on neutrophilic granulocytes may be associated with the interaction of nitric oxide and superoxide radical anions. If the formation of nitric oxide encounters any hindrance, superoxide anion (O -) will activate cells and cause degranulation, thus inducing acute inflammation. Adhesion of neutrophilic granulocyte is an early factor of atherosclerosis. As research shows, nitric oxide prevents formation of atherosclerosis by altering the activity of leukocyte adhesion molecules or inhibiting their expression.

Function of Regulating Growth of Cells

Nitric oxide can inhibit the growth of cells through the following mechanisms: (1) through the interaction with ribonucleotide reductase, inactivating the enzyme so as to inhibit the complex of nucleic acid; (2) affecting the migration of electrons through interaction with cytochrome heme; (3) through altering glyceraldehyde-3-phosphate dehydrogenase and thus damaging glycolysis; (4) reducing the interaction of neutrophilic granulocytes and endothelial cells; (5) inhibiting the adhesion, secretion and aggregation of platelets; (6) increasing the content of intracellular cyclic guanosine monophosphate.

Chapter Four
Say No to Cardio-cerebrovascular Disease

Significance for Discovery and Application of Nitric Oxide

In 2003, throughout the world, about 16.7 million people died of cardio-cerebrovascular disease, accounting for 29.2% of the total mortality. For a long time, it has been viewed that cardio-cerebrovascular disease shows a high incidence in the western countries, but it is now increasing among the population in Asia.

In USA, since 1990, cardio-cerebrovascular disease has been the number one cause of death each year, followed by cancer. The annual mortality caused by cardio-cerebrovascular disease is the total mortality caused by the 7 diseases that follow it. The World Health Organization list of world's top ten causes of death in 2011 includes ischemic heart disease as the first one, for which the mortality rate was 12.8%. Stroke and other cerebrovascular diseases are the second place, with a mortality rate of 10.8%.

In 2010, in Beijing, international research workers presented the latest evidence that research on 500,000 persons in Asia shows, cardio-cerebrovascular disease is starting to constitute a severe threat to the health and wealth of China and other Asian countries and many of the Asian people will be threatened, at their middle age, by heart disease and stroke. The patients of heart disease in Asia are much younger than those in the west. Cardio-cerebrovascular disease is a common disease threatening the health of mankind, especially the middle aged and the elderly. Even if the currently advanced therapy is applied, more than 50% of the survivors of cerebrovascular accidents will not be able to be completely independent. Cardio-cerebrovascular disease results in a high mortality rate, a high disability rate, a high recurrence rate and numerous complications.

Cardiovascular diseases include hypertension, coronary heart disease, myocardial infarction, angina pectoris and so on, while cerebrovascular diseases include such diseases as cerebral thrombosis, cerebral embolism and cerebral hemorrhage. Cardio-cerebrovascular diseases are caused by arteiosclerosis, hypertension, hyperlipidemia, hyperglycemia, blood hyperviscosity and microcirculation disturbance. As research shows, it is observed that nitric oxide can have the effect of keeping vessels clean, preventing strokes and maintaining blood pressure. Nitric oxide can promote the blood circulation throughout the whole body, prevent arteries from aging and hardening, lower blood viscosity, reduce the formation of clots and thrombosis, recover vascular elasticity, lower blood pressure and strengthen cardiac function and thus effectively prevent and cure cardiovascular disease.

The application of nitric oxide technology can effectively improve the status and incidence of cardio-cerebrovascular diseases. As a safer and more reliable therapy, nitric oxide therapy is highly thought of as a treatment for cardio-cerbrovascular diseases throughout the world. As numerous cases indicate, nitric oxide therapy has helped many people to return to a state of vigorous health. In addition, nitric oxide can also effectively prevent strokes.

In 1998, the Nobel Committee awarded the Nobel Prize for Physiology or Medicine for the breakthrough research in nitric oxide. The news published by the committee detailed the important significance of nitric oxide, the miracle molecule. Previously the American Heart Association called the nitric oxide discovery by

Murad's laboratory the greatest discovery in the past century.

Heart: for patients with arteriosclerosis, the ability of endothelial cells to generate nitric oxide declines, but nitric oxide can be supplied by nitroglycerin and other nitro-vasodilators. Currently, the keynote for invention of cardiovascular drugs rests in applying the knowledge of the information molecule, nitric oxide, to develop more effective and more alternative drugs for the treatment of heart diseases.

Lungs: by inhaling low levels of nitric oxide gas, it is possible to treat severe pulmonary conditions and even save patients' lives. For instance, by using nitric oxide, we can lower the pulmonary artery pressure of high-risk premature infants, but since highly-concentrated nitric oxide may be toxic, the dosage is critical.

Cancer: Nitric oxide can be used to kill a series of germs, fungi, mycoplasma and other pathogens. Since nitric oxide can induce the process of apoptosis, scientists are currently experimenting to see if nitric oxide can be used to inhibit growth of tumors.

Sexual dysfunction: nitric oxide causes penile erection by relaxing the vessels in erectile tissues. This principle has been exploited by pharmaceutical companies to develop drugs to treat impotence, for example Sildenafil by Pfizer, better known as

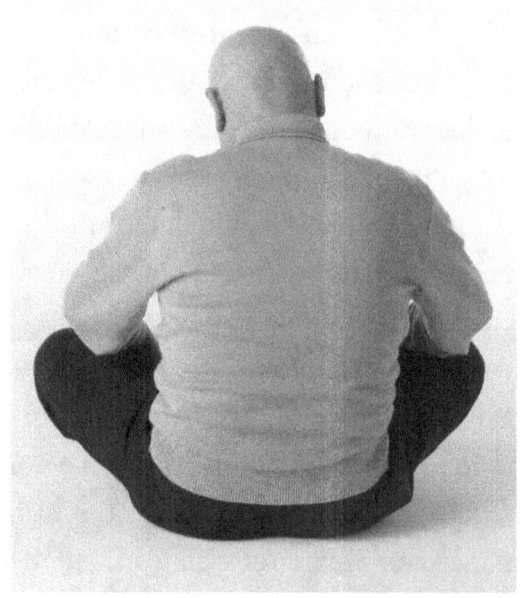

Viagra. Sildenafil can inhibit the enzymatic hydrolysis of cyclic guanosine monophosphate and increase intracellular cyclic guanosine monophosphate due to nitric oxide, so as to maintain the relaxation of vascular smooth muscle and increase blood flow. Viagra has proven effective in combating heart disease and impotence.

Diagnostic analysis: the content of nitric oxide in lung and intestine can be analyzed to monitor inflammatory disease. It can be used in the diagnosis of asthma, colitis and other diseases.

Other functions: nitric oxide plays an important role in olfactory functions and helps in identifying different smells. Additionally, nitric oxide also plays a very important role in our memory.

It is now widely known that nitric oxide plays the role of a signal molecule in the human body and nitric oxide molecules generated in the human body can pass through any cells to reach any tissue in the body. For this reason nitric oxide "signals" can be transmitted from one part of the body to another. Nitric oxide helps to control blood flow to different parts of the human body for vascular dilation to avoid the phenomenon of slow blood flow in vessels, keep vessels clean and open, maintain normal levels of blood pressure and effectively reduce the burden on the heart. In addition, nitric oxide is also an effective weapon against germs, viruses, and various pathogens, and thus significantly protects human health. Therefore, nitric oxide is a "health messenger" in the human body and an important element for human health.

In addition, nitric oxide can regulate the vascular system and blood circulation system of the whole body. When the endothelium issues instructions to the vascular smooth muscle to relax in order to promote blood circulation, it will generate nitric oxide molecules which can easily pass through cell membranes. Upon receipt of this signal, smooth muscle cells around vessels relax. In this way, nitric oxide regulates the vascular system and blood circulation system throughout the whole body and transmits oxygen-containing blood into tissues and organs in order to keep blood pressure stable and nourish tissues. Nitric oxide can also play a role in the neurological system and specific peripheral nerve endings. Through peripheral nerves that release nitric oxide, the brain sends a signal and relaxes the vessels of the penis to facilitate penile erection. In some circumstances, weak erection function is due to a deficiency of nitric oxide generated by nerve endings. "Viagra" can amplify the efficiency of nitric oxide and thus enhance erection.

Nitric oxide molecules generated by the immune system not only can resist the microbes invading the human body, but also can stop, to some extent, the growth of cancer cells and the migration of tumor cells.

PART TWO
PURIFYING HEALTH AT THE SOURCE

It might be difficult to believe that there is a vascular passage in the human body that, if fully extended, could encircle the earth two and a half times. Yet this is the case with blood vessels that make up the human circulation system. We depend on this system not only to transport oxygen and life- giving substances to the various parts of our bodies, but also to discharge waste and refuse, constantly supplementing and purifying our bodies in a complete metabolic cycle. There is no doubt that blood and blood vessels are the keystones of human life and health. One might therefore ask: how can we ensure the health of this life giving system? What effect will vascular aging cause to health? What substances or processes are fundamental to the health of this system? Let us explore the processes on which we all depend to find the answers to these universally important questions.

Chapter One
The Source of Life and Health

Where is the source of health?

Blood can be characterized as a miraculous ever-flowing river. It never stops conveying oxygen and nutritional substances in vessels as well as discharging waste and refuse from inside the human body, repeating the cycle of life. Blood and vessels are the sources of life and health.

In addition to blood itself, the human bloodstream contains numerous nutritional substances, such as inorganic salts, oxygen, cellular metabolites, hormones, enzymes and antibodies, which together perform the functions of providing nutrition to tissues, regulating biological activities and resisting harmful substances.

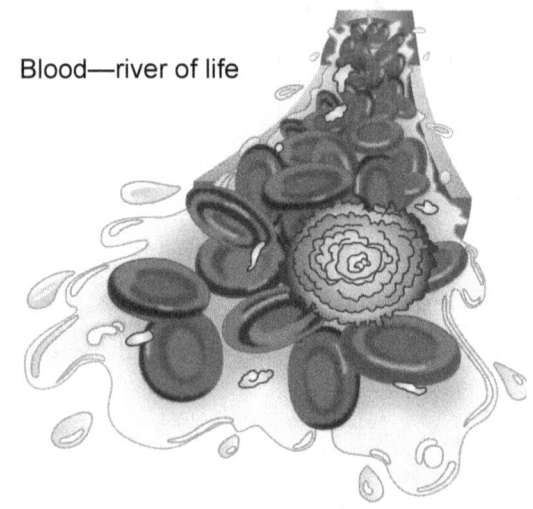

Blood—river of life

The river of blood that flows through each of us, while in one sense familiar, is at the same time highly mysterious to most of us. Yet in the same way that a farmer irrigates his field to ensure the constant growth of healthy crops, so too does blood continually "irrigate" tissues and organs throughout the whole human body, ensuring our health and well-being.

Blood is an opaque red liquid that flows through the heart and through vessels. It accounts for about 8% of the human body weight. In another words, for an adult weighing 60kg, his body will contain about 4800ml of blood, capable of filling several large bottles.

Blood consists of 4 components: plasma, erythrocytes, leukocytes and platelets. Composing about 55% of blood, plasma is a mixture of water, sugar, fat, protein, potassium and calcium, and other substances. Blood cells compose the other 45% of blood. Blood contains different kinds of nutritional components, such as inorganic salt, oxygen, cellular metabolites, hormones, enzymes and antibodies. These substances perform various functions including providing nutrition to tissues, regulating tissue activities and resisting harmful substances.

Functions of blood

To understand the functions of blood, it is necessary to know about the 4 members of the blood "family": erythrocytes, leukocytes, platelets and plasma.

1) Erythrocyte, transporter of oxygen
In the human body, blood plays many roles, but fundamentally, its most important role is one of a substance "transporter". If the circulatory system were a canal, would be the cargo ships, delivering crucial nutrients to their required destinations.
Under a microscope, an erythrocyte has the appearance of a small pie, sagging in the middle, with a diameter of only 7 microns.

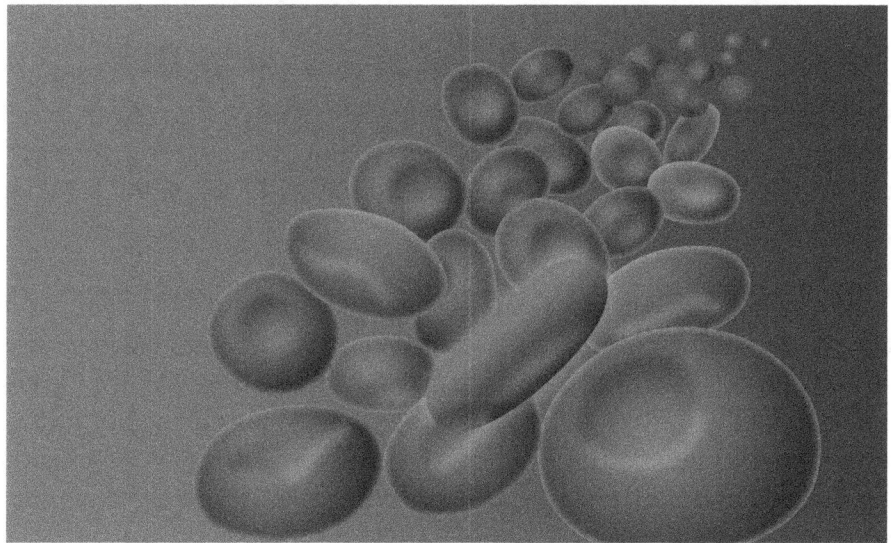

Though small, it conveys oxygen and carbon dioxide (CO_2) to and away from the lungs respectively, resulting in tissue metabolism that ensures normal metabolism within the human body. Additionally, erythrocytes also play a buffering role in acid-alkali balancing. The two functions are achieved with hemoglobin (HB), which is present in all erythrocytes. The condition of anemia can cause erythrocytes to decrease in number or fall in quality, thus affecting the transport function of blood to varying extents and causing a series of pathological changes.

2) Leukocytes, eliminating invaders
Whether in the air, water, or on everyday objects, bacteria and viruses are omnipresent in our daily lives. Were it not for leukocytes, our body would be defenseless against the constant onslaught of microbes on our systems.
Leukocytes are significantly larger than erythrocytes and can move in a similar way to amoebas. They pass through capillaries to enter the surrounding tissues and consume undesirable molecules such as bacteria when they invade the human body. The pus that can often be seen running from an open wound is in fact composed of dead viruses and "sacrificed" leukocytes.

3) Platelets, consolidating the barrier of blood
In blood, platelets are the smallest cells, yet they are absolutely essential members of the blood family. In our life, we cannot avoid getting injured and bleeding from time to time, but as long as vessels are not injured, bleeding will stop automatically as platelets work frantically to stop and seal the wound.

4) Plasma, the maintainer of equilibrium
Apart from such cellular components as erythrocytes, leukocytes and platelets, blood also contains plasma, a kind of light yellow liquid that accounts for 55% of the total volume of blood in the human body. Though not containing any living cells, the role of plasma cannot be ignored in maintaining the stability of the body's internal environment.

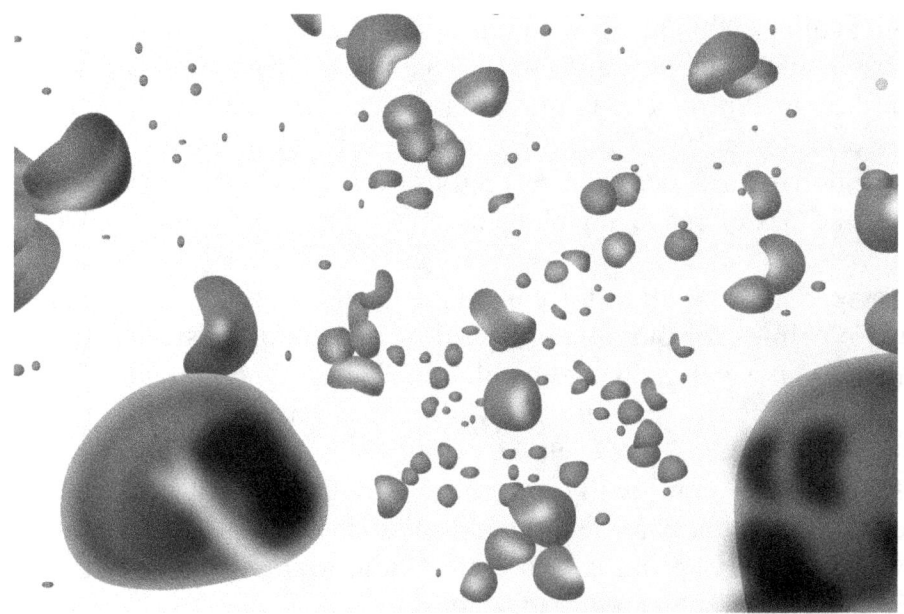

The foodstuffs that we consume and the activities we participate in daily will invariably provoke changes in the body's internal environment, but such changes always occur within a range that our body can bear due to the equilibrium that plasma helps to maintain through colloid osmotic pressure and acid-alkali balancing functions in the blood.

In addition, plasma also plays a role in transporting nutrition and metabolites, as well as participating in the processes of in coagulation and immunization.

Vessels, passage of life

Does blood flow chaotically throughout the body? Obviously not. Blood has pipelines of its own, known as vessels. Vessels refer to a series of channels through which blood flows. Except for the cornea, finger and toe nails, enamel and epithelia, vessels are spread throughout the entire human body. Vessels can be classified into 3 types according to their structure and function: artery, vein and capillary.

The Mississippi River is the world's fourth longest river system, with a length of 6020 km However, it is small in comparison to the blood vessels within the human body , which add up to a total length of 100 million meters -- enough to wind around the Earth two and a half times! Human blood is extremely precious, as it conveys different nutritional substances and oxygen to every part of the human body, and the task of conveying blood itself is completed by the 100,000 km of vessels.

Vessels are a pipeline for conveying blood. Arteries and veins are the pipelines for output and backflow and capillaries are the arena for the physical exchange of blood substances. Arteries and veins are connected by capillaries, while vessels of the whole body are structured as a massive enclosed pipeline. One artery starts at the heart and branches continually, eventually dividing into a huge number of capillaries that are distributed to tissues and cells throughout the whole body. Capillaries integrate again, gradually forming veins before their eventual return to heart.

Classification of Vessels

1) Artery
Artery is a general term for vessels that deliver blood from the heart to different parts of the human body. With the trunk of an artery starting from the left ventricle, the artery branches again and again, its diameter becoming gradually smaller, its vascular wall gradually becoming thinner and its elastic fibers decreasing gradually while smooth muscle tissues assume an increasingly important role. Arteries in the body are structured in a similar fashion to tree branches. The arterial wall is thick, containing three layers; intima, media and adventitia. Media are more developed, containing circular smooth muscle and elastic fiber and adapting to the properties of faster arterial blood flow and higher blood pressure. An artery is divided into three types based on its diameter: large, medium and small. Large arteries have a diameter of 2~3cm; the wall media contains elastic fiber and can bear high pressure; when the ventricle is not pumping blood, the large arterial wall elasticity retracts and plays the role of auxiliary pump. The wall media of a medium artery is developed smooth

muscle, which can cause the lumen to reduce or expand significantly and plays the role of regulating blood volume. Arteries with a diameter of less than 1mm and visible with the naked eye are called small arteries, while the smallest artery has an inner diameter of only 20~30microns, of which the media still has smooth muscle. These arteries carry out systolic-diastolic motion with the beating heart cycle under the control of nerves and chemicals, and regulate blood flow and blood pressure.

Tips:
Pressure change due to heart beating causes the main arterial wall to expand and contract. The peripheral transfer of such beating along the arterial wall is your pulse. Pulse is a characteristic of arteries and the commonly known pulse means a pulse felt on the radial artery in the wrist. The pulse frequency of a normal person is consistent with the heartbeat frequency. In a calm state, an adult has a pulse frequency of 70~75 times per min. Pulse can reflect the state of the blood circulation system and body function, and indicates the beating of the heart and its rhythm.

2) Vein
A vein is a vessel for returning blood to the heart. Veins start by capillaries and end at the atrium in the heart. Blood in systemic veins contains more CO_2 and has a dark red color. Blood in pulmonary veins contains more oxygen and has a fresh red color. Veins start from capillaries, gradually converge to form medium veins and big veins, in the process of returning to heart, and eventually inject into atrium. Human veins are structured as conflux of rivers. As with arteries, venous walls are also divided into intimae, media and adventitia, but are different from arteries in several ways: venous walls have undeveloped media and have less smooth muscle, insignificant elastic fiber and thin walls with less elasticity. Compared to the corresponding arterial vessels, venous vessels have a larger diameter and thin wall, thus have a comparatively big capacity and are easy to expand. At any given time, the human body has about 70% of its blood in the venous system. Changes of vein capacity can have a

great impact on the volume of blood in circulation, so the vein is also known as "capacitance vessel". In most parts of the vein cavity, there are semi-lunar dorsal ruffles, known as venous valves, which prevent the backflow of blood. Veins are classified as deep and shallow veins: a deep vein is accompanied by an artery and a shallow vein is the subcutaneous "blue veins", also known as subcutaneous vein, usually without an artery in companion. Upper and lower extremities have developed veins, which are the ideal places blood transfusion and injection.

3) Capillary

Capillaries are extremely fine vessels, with an average diameter of 6~9microns. They are the most widely distributed vessels in the body and connect arteries to veins. The wall of a capillary is a single layer of cells thick and therefore is highly permeable, allowing it to serve as a place for physical exchange of blood nutrients and tissue substances. In tissues, capillaries have many branches, which are interlinked and anastomosed to form a network. In 0.5mm2 of muscle, there are more than 1,000 capillaries. The total area of human capillary is huge: for a person weighing 60kg, the total area of his/her capillaries will be about 6,000m^2.

Blood circulation: transport line of life

Flow of blood in vessels forms blood circulation, while the circulation system is an enclosed transport system composed of the heart, arteries, veins and capillaries. With the heart beating continuously, power is provided to promote blood to circulate therein, providing different cells present in the body with essential substances, oxygen, nutritional substances and hormones to tissues, and removing tissue refuse so as to ensure the normal metabolism of the human body.

Composition of the human blood circulation system

The human blood circulation system consists of two parts: systemic circulation and pulmonary circulation. Systemic circulation begins

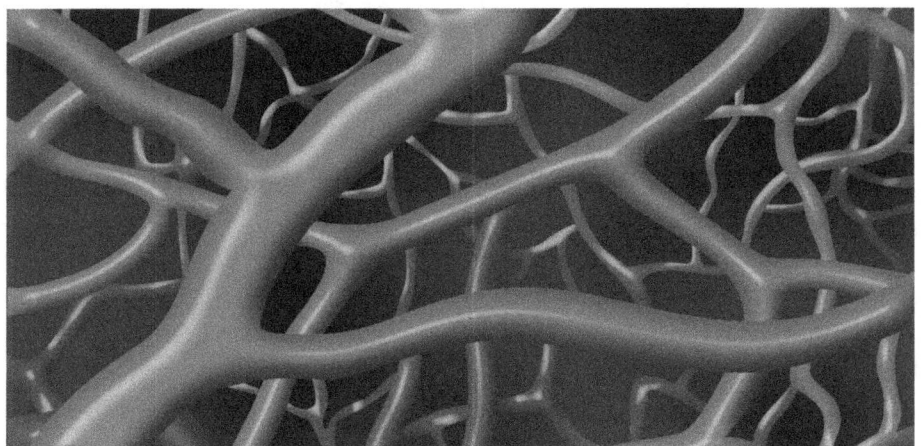

in the left heart ventricle. After it is pumped out of the left ventricle, blood flows through the main artery called the aorta into its derivative arterial branches that send the blood into the relevant organs. The arteries continue to branch several times, with the diameter gradually becoming smaller and number of vessels gradually increasing, before eventually reaching the capillary, where substance exchange takes place with tissue cells. Oxygen and nutritional substances in the blood are absorbed by tissues, while CO_2 and other metabolites in tissues enter the blood, transforming arterial blood into venous blood. Blood returning from the capillaries returns to the heart through the venous system. As the veinous network progresses toward the heart, the venous diameter becomes gradually larger and number of veins dcreases gradually till eventually all the veins gather to the superior vena cava and inferior vena cava vein, from where blood returns to the right atrium, thus completing the process of systemic circulation.

Pulmonary circulation starts in the right ventricle. After it is pumped from the right ventricle, venous blood reaches the capillary net around alveolae in the lung via the pulmonary artery, where it discharges CO_2 and absorbs fresh oxygen, changing from venous blood into arterial blood, before flowing back, via pulmonary veins, into the left atrium. Blood flows from the left atrium into the left ventricle, before circulating throughout the entire body. In this way, with continual systemic circulation and pulmonary circulation, the important task of blood circulation is achieved.

The blood circulation system is composed of two parts: the cardiovascular system and the lymphatic system. The lymphatic system is a support system for the vein system, while the common circulation system means the cardiovascular system.

Blood circulation is the transport line of life, made up of the blood, vessels and heart. It is an enclosed transport system comprising the heart, vessels, capillaries and blood. The heart beats continually to pump blood throughout the body, which provides cells with essential substances (including nutritional substances and oxygen), as well as carrying CO_2, the product of cellular metabolism, away from cells.

Additionally, many hormones and other signal substances are also transported through blood to other organs in order to coordinate in the functions of the whole body. Therefore, maintaining the health of the circulation system is crucial for the survival of the human body, while its core function is to maintain the blood pressure at a normal level. For different tissues and organs of the human body to maintain a normal active life, the heart must beat continually to ensure blood supply. Nevertheless, as a powerful, muscular organ, the heart also needs sufficient nutrition and energy. The vascular system that supplies nutrition to the heart consists of the coronary arteries and veins, also known as coronary circulation. The coronary artery is the artery that supplies blood to the heart, originating from the root of main artery, including the left and right branches, traveling on the surface of heart. Between coronary arteries, there are also abundant anastomosis branches or collateral branches. Though small, the coronary artery has a very large flood flow, accounting for 5% of cardiac output; the amount of blood pumped out of the heart, and ensures the heart has sufficient nutrition to beat powerfully day and night. The Coronary vein works in conjunction with the coronary artery to collect venous blood by merging to the coronary sinus and then the heart's right atrium. In the event that the coronary artery suddenly becomes blocked with a plaque or clot and collateral circulation is not initiated in time, this can lead to myocardial infarction due to a lack of oxygen and nutrients to the heart.

Gradually contaminated source of health

Blood is like a rushing river, conveying oxygen and nutritional substances, irrigating the tissues and organs of the body as well as conveying waste and refuse. Natural aging, unhealthy lifestyles, unhealthy diets, and contaminated environments will cause waste and refuse to accumulate gradually in the body. If they are not promptly cleared and maintained, the river of life will be contaminated and refuse will gradually accumulate inside vessels, causing blood to become turbid and to run slowly. Over time, vessels become narrow and may become blocked. This process can be compared to a contaminated river with a steadily rising river bed, rife with pollutants, or a beaver dam that blocks the flow of a river or stream. The contamination of the blood stream in this way is often so gradual as to be unnoticeable, yet it can be fatally detrimental to human health. How is the blood refuse created? And how can we prevent blood contamination before it takes place?

How is human blood refuse created?

Blood refuse includes two types: one is the exogenous refuse entering into blood from outside; the other is the endogenous refuse created by metabolic activity of human body. Exogenous refuse, also known as uncontrollable refuse, is what we cannot change, while endogenous refuse, also known as controllable blood refuse, is what can be improved by changing our lifestyle or exerting other external influences.

Exogenous refuse

Industrial progress is also accompanied with environmental contamination, which introduces many exogenous refuse into human body. For instance, vegetables, fish and poultry meat that we eat every day are contaminated, to different extents, by such harmful substances as pesticide, fertilizer and hormones. We are living in an environment that is polluted by a huge amount of automobile exhaust, industrial waste gas, heavy metals and dust. Environmental factors are extremely hard for us to change. Nevertheless, nowadays, we are also safeguarding the environment and controlling pollution, but during the course of urban modernization, harm caused by exogenous pollution to the human body is practically unavoidable.

Endogenous refuse

The unhealthy lifestyles of modern humans, includes lack of exercise, and high fat intake, resulting in the dysfunction of our endocrine system and nervous system. As a result, the metabolites and toxins released from tissues and organs in the human body cannot be eliminated and are deposited in blood, and are collectively called endogenous refuse.

Endogenous refuse, also known as controllable blood refuse, can be dealt with by changes in lifestyle or using external factors (such as medicine, healthy diet, etc.).

Reasons for formation of endogenous blood refuse are outlined mainly as follows:

1) Hyperphagia: if one eats too much, the body is unable to digest and absorb all the food, resulting in excess food matter residues. Additionally, for excessive food, digestive organs need to run fully and blood is concentrated in digestive organs, causing the excretory organs to be in a state of dormancy. Intracorporal residues continue to increase and accumulate in the bloodstream as refuse, thus causing blood contamination.

2) Pressure: tension will cause vessels to compress and blood pressure to rise. Other symptoms include cold sweat, a pale complexion and cold hands and feet. Being in such a state for long time will hinder blood flow, and thus cause blood to fail to circulate normally. Just like a river, once water stops flowing, silt in water will be deposited. If blood fails to flow, the refuse in blood will also be deposited in blood vessels.

3) Damp cold: a cold body will not only cause vessels to contract, blood flow to be hindered, and refused to be deposited in the blood, but also the failure to metabolize fat, sugar and refuse.

4) Inadequate motion and unsmooth excretion: inadequate motion will cause muscle to decay and contract, intracorporal heat to decrease and the failure to metabolize refuse in blood, while aggregation of refuse in blood and vessels will also cause contamination.

The harmful effects of blood refuse

When the human body reaches the age of 20, blood refuse gradually starts to be deposited in vessels before eventually changing the vessels into huge "refuse yards". Dark red and thick blood causes vessels to gradually rise like a river bed and forces blood pressure to rise. With blood refuse deposited on the vascular wall, vessels lose their elasticity and become crisp and hard; some plaques form thrombi. When a thrombus blocks cardiac vessels and cerebral vessels, cerebral hemorrhage, cerebral thrombus, and myocardial infarction can take place...... blood refuse not only damages blood cells and vessels, but can also encroach upon cells, tissues and organs in other parts of the human body, cause blood flow velocity to slow down in the human body and vessels to age, resulting in a higher incidence of different lesions and diseases.

According to reports by Information Times, statistics of American College of Cardiology (ACC) suggest cardio-cerebrovascular diseases resulting from blood refuse can cause up to 15 million deaths in the world each year. As one ACC expert pointed out, timely removal of refuse toxins in blood is an effective method for prevention and control. Since blood refuse are the sources for many diseases, removal of blood refuse is a fundamental approach and only short-cut for restoring to health.

As the body ages, the likelihood of disease increases, and the human body will be contaminated even more severely. The ability of the human body to purify blood also decreases with aging, leading to the accumulation of even more toxins. In the US, studies estimate about 80 million people suffer from atherosclerotic plaque; that's roughly 36 percent of the population.

"3 Ls, 3 Hs" harmful effects of blood refuse

Low awareness rate: while most people are generally in a state of reasonable health, they often have no idea until they participate in a medical checkup.

Low cure rate: conditions will get worse without effective treatment upon incidence.

Low controllability rate: blood contamination-related conditions are capable of causing sudden heart failure and even death, which is also hard to prevent and control.

High incidence: there is an extremely high number of people with unhealthy blood in China: it is estimated that the blood of more than one third of people is in an unhealthy state.

High mortality: common causes of death include coronary heart disease, myocardial infarction, cerebral hemorrhage, etc.

High disability: generally a consequence of cerebral hemorrhage and cerebral infarction.

Blood refuse is the source of vascular aging

More than 90% of people do have a low awareness of vascular health. Human vessels will not remain unchanged, but will grow as the human body does, as well as aging naturally as the human body ages. Blood refuse will continue to damage the passage of blood flow: vessels. As we know, rubber hoses for sewage drainage can be easily damaged; the same is true of vessels containing contaminated blood. For instance, when the house tap water pipes and gas pipes are used for long, their inner walls will get scaled and rusty. Gradually, such pipelines are choked and fail to supply water and gas. Similarly for vessels, as the body ages, substances such as cholesterol and triglyceride will accumulate on vascular walls, flexibility in vascular walls declines, vessels harden and blood flow is hindered, eventually causing cardio-cerebrovascular diseases due to ischemia. It is for this reason that we associate cardio-cerebrovascular diseases as well as coronary heart disease and strokes with old age. After blood refuse erodes blood and vessels, vascular damage causes the major organs in the human body to develop symptoms, including acute myocardial infarction, cerebral strokes, renal vascular disease and peripheral vascular disease. Such diseases are not due to lesions of the heart or cerebrum, but rather to atherosclerosis and local obstruction of vessels supplying blood to organs.

World Health Organization data show that cardiovascular disease causes more deaths each year than any other disease. In 2008, an estimated 7.3 million people died of ischemic heart disease, 6.2 million people died of stroke or other cerebrovascular disease. Accounting for 30% of total global deaths.

Blood refuse is the prime culprit causing the blood flow to slow down

The decrease of blood flow velocity in the human body is due to blood refuse. Deposit of refuse in blood and vascular aging will cause blood flow to slow down and even to become blocked; consequently, blood cannot flow smoothly and is hindered in supplying nutrition to tissues and organs in the human body, resulting in a higher incidence of various diseases.

Just as the name implies, blood flow velocity decrease means that being blocked in vessels, blood fails to flow normally, as is known as "blocked blood flow" in Europe and America. Vessels are elastic and their inner walls are very soft for the purpose of keeping blood flowing smoothly. As age increases and bad habits remain, lipids are deposited on the vascular wall intimae, especially cholesterol and other blood refuse, resulting in uneven intimal surfaces. Sometimes, uneven vascular cavities are accompanied by calcium deposits and fiber formation. If the vessels of such lesions could be seen as a cross section, it would be possible to observe that cholesterol deposits are just like off-white atheromatous plaques. Obviously, as vascular wall intimae become thicker and fiber and calcium are deposited, vessels also become hard and passages on the inner wall of vessels become increasingly narrow, resulting in unsmooth blood flow.

All parts of the human body may experience the phenomenon of blood flow slowdown. As parts with blood flow velocity slowing increase, blood runs increasingly slowly in vessels, and human tissues and organs fail to receive blood and nutrition in time; ischemia of tissues and organs, unsmooth blood flow, and inadequate delivery of nutritional components and oxygen cause functional decay and necrosis to different extents, resulting in great inconvenience and pain in daily life and even life-threatening illnesses. The phenomena of blood flow velocity slowdown is widely observed in middle-aged and older people, and has shown a growing tendency in recent years. Due to their prevalence in many people and severity, such phenomena have attracted much attention in medical circles.

Chapter Two
Harmful effects of Blood Flow Slowdown

Hazards of cardio-vascular blood flow slowdown

Heart supplies blood to the whole body. Does the heart also need to be serviced by blood?

For tissues and organs of the human body to maintain their normal functions, the heart is required to beat continuously to ensure blood supply. As a muscular power organ pumping blood, the heart itself also requires sufficient nutrition and energy. The vascular systems that supply nutrition to heart are the coronary artery and vein, and are known collectively as coronary artery circulation. If blood flow velocity slows down in coronary circulation, the heart will fail to work normally due to lack of sufficient nutrition and will lead to coronary heart disease, myocardial infarction, etc.

Hazards of cerebral-vascular blood flow velocity slowing

There are two pairs of vessels supplying cerebral blood: one is the internal carotid arteries, comprising the internal carotid arterial system; the other is the vertebral arteries, comprising the vertebralbasilar arterial system.

Internal carotid arterial system: on the left and right sides of neck, there is one massive artery known as common carotid artery, the beat of which we can feel by hand. The artery branching from the common carotid artery into the skull is called the internal carotid artery. This artery is divided, into five main branches upon entering the skull: the anterior cerebral artery, the middle cerebral artery, the ocular artery, the posterior communicating artery and anterior choroidal artery, all of which together supply three fifths of blood for ocular and the anterior cerebral hemisphere, including the temporal lobes, the parietal lobes and the basal ganglia area.

Vertebralbasilar arterial system: vertebral arteries begin at the subclavian artery, with one branch on left and right respectively, running through five transverse foraminae on both sides of cervical vertebrae; upon rising into the skull through the foramen magnum, the two vertebral arteries converge at the anterior cerebral lower margin to form the large basilar artery, all of which is collectively known as the vertebralbasilar arterial system. When it reaches the midbrain area, the basilar artery is in turn divided into two posterior cerebral arteries, supplying 2/5 of posterior cerebral blood, including occipital lobe, basal surface of temporal lobe and thalamus. Branches of vertebralbasilar artery at the cerebellum and pontine supply blood to the cerebellum and pontine artery systems. The two anterior cerebral arteries are linked with the anterior communicating branch artery, while the two collateral internal carotid arteries are linked with the posterior cerebral artery by the posterior communicating branch artery, forming the cerebral artery Circle of Willis. When blood flow is blocked at any part of the Circle of Willis, supply can be regulated by adjusting access from different points. Additionally, internal carotid artery can also be anastomosed with facial, maxillary, temporal and other arteries through the ocular artery. The vertebral artery can also be anastomosed with arteries on the surface of the brain in various directions, while collateral branch circulation is abundant. Thus, there are considerable alternatives for blood flow to some parts of the brain. The cerebrum has extremely abundant arteries which are also highly sensitive to hypoxia. If blood circulation in cerebrum stops for

3~4min, the human body will lose consciousness; if blood circulation stops for 4~5 minutes, there is a 50% chance of permanent cerebral damage; if it stops for 10 minutes, though not being completely damaged, cognitive abilities will be severely damaged. This is why cerebrovascular diseases incur a high rate of disability.

Hazards of blood flow slowdown of vessels in periosteum

Periosteum is hard connective tissue capsule covered by bone surface except for the joints. At the parts where tendons are adhered, periosteum adheres very closely to bones. In parts, periosteum is thick and can be easily stripped off from bones. Periosteum consists of two parts, the outer layer of which is formed of combinations of collagen fibers, rich with vessels to provide nutrition to skeleton.

If vessels in periosteum are observed to have blood flow slowdown, it will result in skeletal malnutrition and cause such diseases as in femoral head necrosis, joint aging and degrading, rheumatism and arthralgia.

Hazards of blood flow slowdown in vessels in the reproductive system

Such diseases as arterial atherosclerosis, arterial damage, artery stenosis, pudendal artery bypass and abnormal cardiac function are all likely to result in the reduction of arterial blood flow in the corpus cavernosum. Reduced blood flow to the genitals will cause difficulty in achieving sexual arousal (in both male and female bodies).

Hazards of blood flow slowdown in the circulation system.

Poor circulation in extremities that causes cold hands and feet is closely associated with poor cardiac and vascular health, as blood is pumped from the heart and is transmitted, together with oxygen, to different parts of the human body. Metabolizing nutrients will produce heat so that the hands and feet can stay warm. Once the cardiovascular system fails and blood cannot be delivered extremities in the body, hands and feet will become cold.

Chapter Three
Preventive Measures for Health

How to check to see if your blood is healthy

Changes in lifestyle, working pressure, nutritional intake and environmental hygiene levels are all capable of influencing the health of our blood. The resulting physiological metabolic disorders will result in lipid abnormality, diabetes, hypertension, anemia, etc. Such blood is called "unhealthy blood".

Using the following tests, you can check if your blood is healthy or contaminated. Please answer "Yes" or "No" to the following points.

○ Dizziness, chest pain, palpitation, chest distress: Yes/No

○ Pale cheeks, dizziness and dim eyesight, lassitude, fatigue and physical weakness: Yes/No

○ Thirst, low urine output, weight loss: Yes/No

○ Severe headaches: Yes/No

○ Crispy nails, dry yellow hair: Yes/No

○ Failure to curb harmful habits (smoking, drinking, eating sweet food): Yes/No

○ Lack of exercise in daily life: Yes/No

○ Bruising for unknown reason: Yes/No

○ Lack of vegetables and fruit in diet: Yes/No

○ Suffering from any chronic disease: Yes/No

○ Living in the area with higher than average radiation levels : Yes/No

● In case of "Yes" for less than 2 items, it means a mild blood contamination.

● In case of "Yes" for 2~5 items, it will bemoderate blood contamination.

● In case of "Yes" for more than 5 items, it will severe blood contamination, to which much attention shall be given.

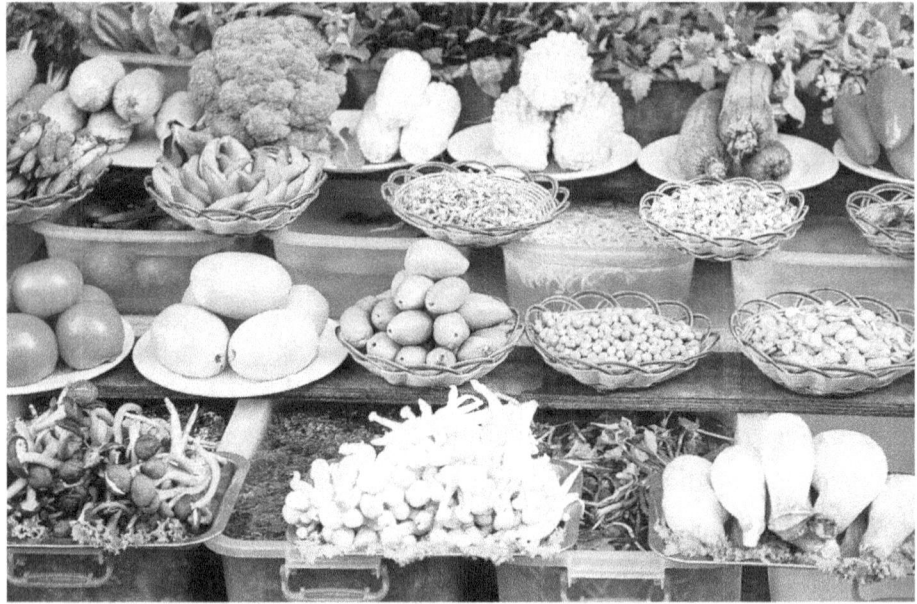
Lack of vegetables and fruit in diet will affect the health of blood

How to detect whether vessels are healthy

1) Assess the vascular age by the state of health

Emotionally depressed recently? Often forgetful? Feeling a chest pain when climbing stairs? ......If the answers to these questions are all affirmative, it is the time to pay attention to your "vascular age".

By knowing about the physiological functions of vessels and hazards of vascular diseases, one can understand the importance of keeping vessels "young" to ensuring a long and healthy life. Therefore, it is important to conduct a self-assessment of your vascular age to make the necessary adjustments to lifestyle in time and keep vessels young and healthy. Foreign experts have proposed the following self-assessment procedure for vascular age:

○ Emotionally depressed: Yes/No
○ Excessively conscientious: Yes/No
○ Fond of eating instant noodles, biscuits and refreshments: Yes/No
○ Preference for meat: Yes/No
○ Unwilling to go to the playground: Yes/No
○ Cigarettes smoked daily multiplied by age exceeding 400: Yes/No
○ Chest pain when climbing stairs: Yes/No
○ Cold hands and feet, with a sense of numbness: Yes/No
○ Poor memory and frequent forgetfulness: Yes/No
○ Blood pressure increase: Yes/No
○ Cholesterol or blood glucose rise: Yes/No
○ Relatives who have died of coronary heart disease or stroke: Yes/No
○ If you answered "Yes" for 1~4 items, it indicates that your vessels are still young and that you should try to maintain your current health level.
● If you answered "Yes" for 5~7 items, it indicates your vascular age is 10 years older than your physiological age.
● If you answered "Yes" for 8~12 items, it indicates your vascular age is 20 years older than your physiological age.

The latter two circumstances should prompt you seriously to reconsider aspects of your lifestyle.

2) Assess the symptoms of "sticky blood" by examining the state of your health
Using the following body "signals", you can detect the symptoms of sticky blood. Answer the following questions using "Yes" or "No".
○ Feeling tight at chest and neck: Yes/No
○ Blackened complexion and flushed face: Yes/No
○ Blackened lips: Yes/No
○ Blackened gums: Yes/No
○ Dark skin: Yes/No
○ Easily bruised: Yes/No
○ Flushing palms: Yes/No
○ Cobweb vessels in chest area: Yes/No

○ Frequent oral ulcers: Yes/No
○ Sometimes feeling weak when climbing stairs: Yes/No
○ Numbness in legs and feet when walking, which will disappear after a rest: Yes/No
○ Palpitations: Yes/No
○ Occasional cardiac arrhythmia: Yes/No
○ Cramping legs: Yes/No
○ Anxiety: Yes/No
○ Feeling cold: Yes/No
○ Occasionally feeling shoulder, knee or back pain: Yes/No
○ Male: ED (Erectile dysfunction): Yes/No
○ Female: Amenorrhoea: Yes/No
● If you answered "Yes" for more than 7 items, there is a severe risk of sticky blood.
● If you answered "Yes" for more than 5 items, there is a danger of risk blood.
● If you answered "Yes" for more than 3 items, there is a moderate risk of potential sticky blood.
● If you answered "Yes" for less than 2 items, there are no significant problems with your blood.

3) Assess vascular aging by living habits
The following body "signals" may indicate vascular aging. Answer the checking points by "Yes" or "No".
○ Drinking two bottles of beer daily: Yes/No
○ Almost no time for exercising: Yes/No
○ Eating deserts daily: Yes/No
○ Feeling high pressure: Yes/No
○ Preference for eating meat: Yes/No
○ Smoking: Yes/No
○ Preference for vehicle transport rather than walking: Yes/No
○ Lack of sleep related to anxiety: Yes/No
○ Waist measures more than 85cm for male and 90cm for female: Yes/ No
○ Eating bread with large quantities of butter: Yes/No
○ Taking exercise previously but stopped now: Yes/No

○ Fond of taking a hot bath: Yes/No
○ Fond of eating greasy food or fast food or other unhealthy snacks: Yes/No
○ Preference for relatively sweet drinks: Yes/No
○ Weight increase of more than 5kg compared to when you are most slim: Yes/No
○ Prefer to use elevator rather than stairs: Yes/No
○ Seldom eat vegetables: Yes/No
○ Frequently waking up at midnight: Yes/No
● If you answered "Yes" for more than 7 items, there may be a high risk of vascular aging.
● If you answered "Yes" for more than 5 items, there may be a risk of vascular aging.
● If you answered "Yes" for more than 3 items, there is a moderate risk of vascular aging.
● If you answered "Yes" for less than 2 items, vessels are still young and healthy.

Chapter Four
A Purifying Agent as the Source of Health

The health of blood and vessels is the foundation of human health as a whole. Yet it is only when people experience physical problems that they begin to pay attention to this aspect of their well-being. Even when problems arise, there is a tendency for individuals to assume that problems can be dealt with by taking a few vitamins. However, to ensure the health of our circulatory system, only nitric oxide can help us to take effective measures against blood related conditions before they arise, to prevent the formation of refuse in our blood vessels.

Keep blood and vessels healthy

Thanks to their small molecular weight and being lipophilic, nitric oxide can penetrate any cell to reach any tissue, and is the only "messenger" that simultaneously qualifies as an intracellular and extracellular messenger molecule. It can travel through all the tissues and organs of the human body, and can quickly repair damaged vascular endothelial cells, relax vessels, deliver oxygen and nutrition to cells, prevent the phenomenon of blood flow slowdown in vessels, keep vessels clean and smooth, maintain a normal blood pressure, and keep physical functions in normal operation.

When the human body reaches the age of 25~30 years, the secretion of nitric oxide is at its peak; any older and the production of nitric oxide in the human body declines gradually; at age of about 40, those with severely inadequate secretion of nitric oxide will show the significant symptom of "3H". Therefore, the most effective method for maintaining and protecting the health of blood and vessels is to supplement nitric oxide for the human body from the age of about 30.

Avoid the dangers of blood flow slowdown

Nitric oxide is important to ensuring that blood flows smoothly. By expanding vessels, clearing attachments of vascular inner wall, repairing the damaged endothelia of vessels, and clearing blood refuse, it maintains the effective circulation of blood throughout different organs and prevents a series of problems with the human body that occur due to blood flow slowdown.

Preventing the formation of thrombus

Nitric oxide exists in the cardiovascular system, nervous system and throughout the whole body. As it passes through cell membranes, it can deliver specific information or biological signals to regulate cell activity and guide the body as it fulfills a particular function. Among the various roles of nitric oxide, vasodilatation is one of the most important, as this helps to regulate blood flow and keep blood flowing to every part of the human body. Nitric oxide can relax vessels to ensure adequate blood supply to the heart and prevents the formation of thrombus, a condition that causes strokes and heart injury.

Prevention of artery atherosclerosis

Gradual increase of cholesterol and fat inside the coronary artery will result in arteriosclerotic plaques, causing arteries to become narrow and even blocked, thus reducing blood supply to the heart.

One important role of nitric oxide is to slow down the deposit of atherosclerotic plaques on vascular walls, and eliminate such plaques. Since blood and vessels are both of crucial importance to human health, it is essential to avoid diseases and to pursue lifestyle habits that prolong longevity. We can do this by keeping blood healthy and clean and keep vessels young and full of elasticity. Since discovering the properties of nitric oxide, we have achieved a more profound understanding about the source of blood flow-related diseases. Playing a crucial role in the blood circulation system of the human body, nitric oxide can keep blood and vessels healthy and eliminate hazards of blood flow slowdown so that blood flows more smoothly, prevents formation of thrombus and prevents artery atherosclerosis. In other words, nitric oxide is a highly effective "purifying agent" that travels through the life stream of the human body.

PART THREE
THE AMAZING PROPERTIES OF THE MIRACLE MOLECULE

As a messenger, nitric oxide is involved in the execution of various functions such as inflammatory response, signal delivery, vascular regulation and immune system regulation. Nitric oxide is broadly and intimately involved with the physiological functions and the clinical pathology of the digestive system, and, has many functions perhaps including, the development of cancers. Although state of mind, unlike the physical body, cannot be seen nor touched, it directly influences the amount of enzyme and activity of NOS in the body. Patients' psychological status influences their quality of life, and may also have a significant impact on their physical status, including cardiovascular health. The psychological status such as calmness of the mind raises nitric oxide levels in the human body, whilst anger and fear reduce nitric oxide levels. It is important to maintain a good psychological state to keep nitric oxide levels high; for longevity and enhanced quality of life.

Chapter One
Sources and Hazards of "3H"

Many individuals of advanced years will no doubt be intimately familiar with the "3H" conditions (hypertension, hyperlipemia and hyperglycemia), any one of which can cause them to feel uneasy even when eating or sleeping. Nevertheless, the three are inseparable: any one of them may be accompanied by the other two. It may therefore be asked: since any one of these is already terrifying, why are these conditions invariably inflicted on us all at once? Do they have one source?

The answer is simple: vascular aging and blood flow slowdown are the source of the three. When a person is young and vigorous, blood flows smoothly, vessels are adequately elastic and body is naturally healthy, without any blockage, viscosity or deposits. However, as one gets older, refuse will gradually build in the blood causing blood to become sticky and blockage to occur, aging and even rupturing vessels. For instance, for a person aged 20, his blood is bright red, but at the age of 40, blood becomes dark red, as a direct result of the deposit of refuse in the human body that contaminates blood.

World Health Organization data show that the deaths attributed globally to non-communicable diseases, the main risk factors for high blood pressure, accounting for 16.5% of global deaths, followed by tobacco use 9%, hyperglycemia 6%, lack of exercise 6% and 5% overweight and obesity. Hyperlipemia may cause vascular embolization, hypertension may cause cerebral hemorrhage and cerebrovascular strokes, and hyperglycemia may cause diabetes. As the WHO itself clearly states, the first defense line for prevention of cardiovascular diseases is to reduce and control "3H".

Similarly, in a human body at the age of 25~30 years, secretion of nitric oxide is at its peak; any older, and the capacity to produce nitric oxide in the human body declines gradually; at the age of about 40, those with severely inadequate secretion of nitric oxide will show the main symptoms of "3H".

Hypertension

Hypertension is the most common cardiovascular disease in the world as well as one of the biggest epidemic diseases, and often causes complications of such organs as the heart, brain and kidney, severely damaging human health in the process. Therefore, it is of extreme importance to the early prevention and timely treatment that we enhance our understanding of hypertension.

Blood pressure refers to lateral pressure on vascular walls that occurs as a result of bloodflow through vessels. Hypertension is a disease that can be characterized by increased arterial pressure. It is measured with a numerical value using a blood pressure cuff and sphygmomanometer placed at the brachial artery, which is known as BP (blood pressure) value with mmHg or kPa as the unit. The two widely known types of blood pressure are systolic blood pressure (SBP) and diastolic blood pressure (DBP). Systolic blood pressure refers to the lateral pressure of blood on vascular wall when heart is in contraction, while diastolic blood pressure refers to the lateral pressure on the vascular wall when the heart is relaxed. When a doctor records blood pressure, if it is 120/80mmHg, 120mmHg is the systolic blood pressure and 80mmHg is the diastolic blood pressure. To be expressed as per international unit kPa, 1mmHg=0.133kPa, and 120/80mmHg equals to 16/10.6kPa.

According to the blood pressure criteria proposed by the World Health Organization (WHO) to indicate a normal level of health in an adult human body, systolic blood pressure should be lower than or equal to 140mmHg (18.6kPa) and diastolic blood pressure should be lower than or equal to 90mmHg (12kPa). If an adult's systolic blood pressure is higher than or equal to 160mmHg (21.3kPa) and diastolic blood pressure is higher than or equal to 95mmHg (12.6kPa), this indicates hypertension; if the BP value is between the above two, i.e., systolic blood pressure is 141~159mmHg (18.9~21.2kPa) and diastolic blood pressure is 91~94mmHg (12.1~12.5kPa), this also indicates early hypertension. In diagnosing hypertension, it is necessary to measure blood pressure several times; hypertension can be confirmed only when the mean value of DBP for two consecutive times is at or above 90mmHg (12kPa). Any increase in pressure can not be confirmed by one measurement alone.

Hazards of hypertension

Impact of high-pressure blood flow on arterial walls over a long period of time will result in mechanical damage to artery intimae and cause blood lipids to be deposited on arterial walls, forming fat plaques that result in atherosclerosis, arterial stenosis and blood flow blockage.

Additionally, hypertension may also lead to cardiac hypertrophy, heart failure, cardiac angina and myocardial infarction; long-term hypertension will result in ventricular dilatation, resulting in hypertension cardiomyopathy. After cardiac hypertrophy and heart failure, cardiac pumping function is irregular, causing a slowdown of blood flow.

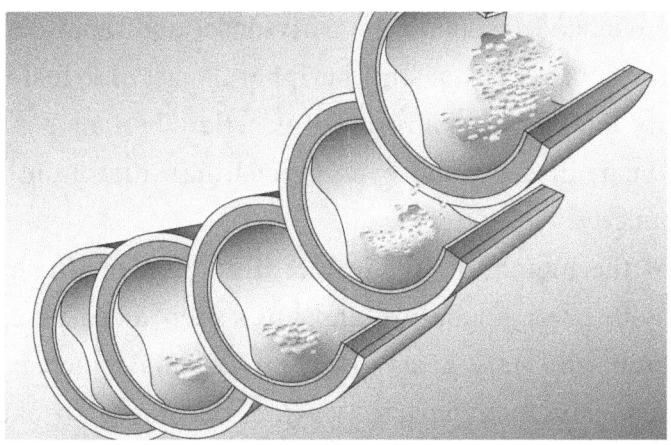

Long-time impact of high-pressure blood flow (with lipids depositing on arterial walls under long-time impact of hypertension)

Hyperlipemia

Abnormal fat metabolism or consumption causes one or more of the lipids present in plasma to be present in levels that are higher than normal, also known as hyperlipemia. Hyperlipemia will cause levels of cholesterol (TC) or triglyceride (TG) in blood to become excessively high, while high-density lipoprotein cholesterol (HDL -C), "the good cholesterol" will become excessively low.

Lipid abnormality is closely associated with various diseases such as obesity, Type II diabetes mellitus, hypertension, coronary heart disease, and cerebral strokes. Long-term lipid abnormality may lead to artery atherosclerosis and increased incidence of potentially fatal cardio-cerebrovascular diseases. As living standards have risen and lifestyles have changed in China, the prevalence of lipid abnormality has also risen significantly. Prevention and control of lipid abnormality is a matter of utmost importance for prolonging and improving the quality of life.

Deposit of lipids in the vascular endothelium leads to artery atherosclerosis and results in the early-onset and rapid development of cardio-cerebrovascular and peripheral vascular lesions. Lipid abnormality that arises as a result of genetic inheritance may initiate coronary heart disease, and even myocardial infarction before the onset of puberty.

As part of the metabolic syndrome, lipid abnormality may often co-exist with or occur before and after such diseases as obesity, hypertension, coronary heart disease, abnormal glucose tolerance or diabetes. Severe hypertriglyceridemia may also cause acute pancreatitis.

The damage of such a condition to the human body is largely concealed, gradual, progressive and systemic. One of the most direct manifestations of the harm it causes is the acceleration of systemic artery atherosclerosis, as the each major organ depends on arteries for blood supply and oxygen supply; once arteries are blocked by atheromatous plaque, the consequences are severe. Such diseases caused by atherosclerosis as renal failure are all closely associated with hyperlipemia. As comprehensive study data show, hyperlipemia is an independent but important hazard for cerebral stroke, coronary heart disease, myocardial infarction, and sudden cardiac death.

The major damage caused by hyperlipemia is the artery atherosclerosis that it results in, which itself leads to numerous related diseases, of which the most common fatal disease is coronary heart disease. Severe chylomicrons may lead to acute pancreatitis, another fatal disease.

In addition, hyperlipemia is a key contributing factor in the development of hypertension, abnormal glucose tolerance and diabetes. Hyperlipemia may also lead to fatty liver, hepatic cirrhosis, cholelithiasis, pancreatitis, brain hemorrhage, peripheral vascular diseases, lameness, and hyperuricemia.

Normal value of blood lipids

Total cholesterol (adults): 2.9—6.0mmol/L

Triglyceride: 0.56—1.7mmol/L

Low-density lipoprotein cholesterol: approximately 2.7mmol/L High-density lipoprotein cholesterol: 0.90—1.55mmol/L

Hazards of hyperlipemia

With a huge amount of "refuse" in blood of hyperlipemia patients, blood becomes sticky, blood flow slows and the vascular endothelium will become damaged over a long period of time, causing endothelium to become unsmooth.

Vascular endothelial damage is often a catalyst for cardio-cerebrovascular diseases. Human vascular endothelium can be compared to the bank of a river; if the bank is smooth and solid, river water can flow by smoothly; if it is not solid, erosion will cause it to collapse, resulting in leakage and river blockage, as well as flooding. The surface of vascular endothelhium in patients with hyperlipemia tends to be uneven, while the connection of vascular endothelial cells gradually loosens. In blood, rising lipids and agglutinating platelets become attached, through endothelial cells, to the uneven vascular walls and gradually form atherosclerosis plaques, affecting blood flow to the heart and cerebrum. The turbulence of the flow of blood increases the amount of atherosclerosis. After the vascular endothelium is damaged, the elasticity of vessels will also deteriorate and vascular spasms can occasionally be observed, thus affecting blood supply to the heart and cerebrum result in various cardio-cerebrovascular diseases. Lipid-reduction, anticoagulation and proper protection of vascular endothelium is the class-I level prevention method for cardio-cerebrovascular diseases.

Hyperglycemia

Hyperglycemia means that glucose levels in the blood are significantly higher than normal, and many who develop this condition may not be aware that they have done so. Hyperglycemia can develop over a period of several days or even several hours. It is defined as a level of glucose in the blood which is higher than 7.8mmol/L. The normal level of glucose in the blood of a person who has not eaten any sugar or food containing sugar for a period of 8 hours is 3.9~6.1mmol/L. Rising glucose levels in the blood and urine may initiate osmotic diuresis and cause symptoms of polyuria, and can also result in increased plasma osmolality when combined with a significant loss of water content. High blood osmolarity may stimulate the thirst center hypothalamus, thus resulting in symptoms such as thirst and polydipsia. Due to relative or absolute lack of insulin, in vivo glucose cannot be utilized, and protein and fat consumption increases, thus causing weight loss. To compensate for the loss of sugar and to maintain body activity, it is necessary to injest more food, resulting in the typical symptoms of eating more, drinking more and urinating more and becoming emaciated. The symptoms of diabetic patients such as polydipsia and polyuria are proportional to the severity of the illness.

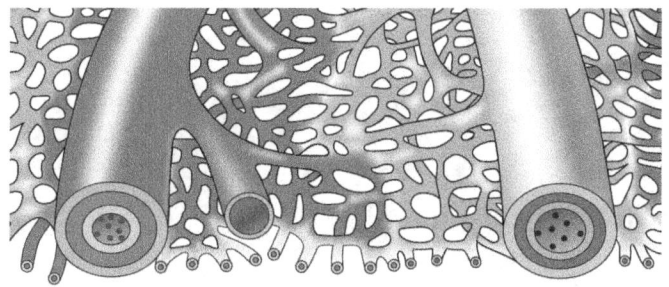

Capillary vessel (the capillary vessel of diabetic patients had thickened)

Hazards of hyperglycemia

Vascular lesions caused by diabetes are associated closely with glucose metabolism and common glycosylation and lipid metabolism abnormality. Diabetic patients typically experience fat metabolism disorder, high lipid levels, fast artery atherosclerosis and slow blood flow. In addition, capillary walls in diabetic patients are often thick, and they suffer from narrowing of the lumen arteries for erythrocytes to pass through and hypoxia of tissues and cells. Therefore, long-term hyperglycemia will cause lesions to all tissues and organs of the whole body, resulting in incidence of acute and chronic complications, such as pancreatic function failure, water loss, electrolyte disorder, malnutrition, lower resistance to disease, renal function damage, nervous lesion, and fundus disease. It is therefore imperative to control hyperglycemia. The high glucose levels in the blood complex with vascular and tissue proteins to decrease their function. The complexes are called "advanced glycosylation end products or AGES". Glycosylation of blood hemoglobin can be used to monitor a patient's treatment of their diabetes.

Chapter Two
Nitric Oxide and "3H"

Coronary heart disease and "3H"

Coronary heart disease is one of the major diseases affecting human health. Using the biomedical model, the disease may be described as clinical angina pectoris or myocardial infarction, even death, resulting from coronary stenosis or occlusion due to the formation of atheromatous plaque in the coronary artery and its subsequent plaque rupture, as well as the formation of thrombus. For some time, various types of drugs for treating angina pectoris have been marketed as well as more interventional measures and bypass surgeries for coronary arteries have been introduced as a treatment, saving many patients from the damaging effects coronary heart disease. However, as a whole, as epidemic factors are effectively controlled, the incidence of coronary heart disease increases sharply year by year, while its lethality and disability also increase sharply, causing an unbearable burden on man and society. Therefore, it is necessary not only to treat the condition medically, but also to draw the attention of the public.

To examine this issue in greater depth, it is necessary to deal with the source of coronary heart disease such as harmful lifestyle habits at an early stage, thereby preventing the damaging effects of hyperlipemia, hypertension, and hyperglycemia. In this way, we can bring down the incidence of coronary heart disease as a whole.

Nitric oxide and hypertension

Primary hypertension is a complication the main clinical manifestation of which is high blood pressure, accompanied or not by various cardiovascular risk factors. Hypertension can cause various cardio-cerebrovascular diseases, affecting the structure and function of important organs such as the heart, brain and kidney and eventually leading to the functional failure of these organs. For this reason, hypertension can often be fatal, and is viewed as a silent but fatal disease if not treated.

Increases in blood pressure over a long period time, catecholamine, angiotension II and other factors can all stimulate myocardial cell hypertrophy and interstitial fibrosis. Hypertension manifests itself mainly as left ventricular hypertrophy and dilatation; according to the extent of left ventricular hypertrophy and dilatation, it can be classified as symmetrical hypertrophy, asymmetrical septal hypertrophy and dilated hypertrophy. When long-term hypertension results in cardiac hypertrophy or dilatation, it is called hypertension cardiopathy. Hypertension cardiopathy is often complicated by coronary artery atherosclerosis and microangiopathy and eventually can lead to heart failure or severe arrhythmia, and even sudden death. Impact of long-term hypertension on brain tissues, such as cerebral stroke or chronic cerebral ischemia, is in fact a consequence ofcere brovas culardisease. Long-term hypertension causes cerebrovascular ischemia and degeneration, promoting cerebral artery atherosclerosis, and atheromatous plaque rupture may be complicated by the formation of cerebral thrombus.

Long-term sustained hypertension causes pressure to rise in the renal glomerular internal capsule. Hypertension also causes glomerular fibrosis and atrophy, and renal atherosclerosis, thus leading to renal essential ischemia and continual reduction of renal function. Chronic renal failure is one of serious consequences of long-term hypertension, especially if complicated by diabetes. In the event of any malignant hypertension, afferent glomerular arteriole and interlobular artery with proliferative intimitis and fibrinoid necrosis may show renal failure after a period of time.

Spasms can be observed in the retinal arterioles in the early stages of hypertension and sclerosis can occur as the disease develops. A sharp rise of blood pressure may lead to retinal exudation and hemorrhage. Vascular endothelial dependent diastolic dysfunction can be observed in hypertensive patients. This is related to a reduction in nitric oxide from vascular endothelial synthesis and the release and increase of active oxygen species or "free radicals". Nitric oxide reduction and active oxygen species increase and play an important role in vascular endothelial dependent diastolic dysfunction in hypertension. Nitric oxide plays a role in relaxing vessels, inhibiting the proliferation of smooth muscular cells and aggregation of platelets, reducing leukocyte adhesion, reducing endothelial cell injury, and preventing the formation of artery atherosclerosis.

By activating soluble guanylate cyclase (sGC), nitric oxide promotes the generation of cyclic guanosine monophosphate (cGMP). As the second critical messenger responsible for regulating multiple physiological processes, cGMP can activate cGMP-dependent protein kinase, causing a decrease in Calcium ion concentration in cytoplasm and calcium influx will be suppressed. Subsequently calcium ion concentration will decrease, and relax smooth muscle within the blood vessel; thereby to reduce blood pressure.

Additionally, nitric oxide helps to clear the refuse that becomes attached to vascular inter walls and promptly repair vascular endothelium, as well as preventing free radicals from attacking the damaged vascular endothelium, so as to protect vessels and restore their elasticity.

Nitric oxide and hyperlipemia

Blood lipid is a general term for neutral fat (triglyceride and cholesterol) in plasma and lipids (phospholipid, glycolipid, sterol). Plasma lipoprotein is a spherical macromolecular complex consisting of protein [apoprotein (apo)] triglyceride, cholesterol, and phospholipid. With the ultracentrifugation method, plasma lipoprotein can be classified into 5 major groups: chylomicron (CM); Very-Low-Density Lipoprotein (VLDL); Intermediate-Density Lipoprotein (IDL); Low-Density Lipoprotein (LDL) and High-Density Lipoprotein (HDL). The buoyant density of such 5 lipoproteins increases in this sequence.

Nitric oxide can inhibit the synthesis of LDL, causing the quantitative reduction of LDL in blood in a short period of time as well as a corresponding reduction in blood of cholesterol and triglycerides (TG). Additionally, nitric oxide can promote the synthesis of HDL, causing cholesterol and TG in blood to be rapidly conveyed out of the blood vessels to the liver for the purpose of metabolizing, excreting and reducing lipid levels.

Nitric oxide and hyperglycemia

Diabetes is a set of metabolic diseases characterized by a chronic increase of blood glucose (glucose for short) level that is initiated by insulin secretion and functional defects. It may lead to chronic progressive changes, function deterioration and failure of tissues and organs such as the eye, kidney, nerve, heart and vessels. In case of severe illness or stress, severe metabolic disorder may occur. Diabetes is a common and frequent disease, the prevalence of which is rapidly rising with improvement of people's living standards, an aging population and changes in lifestyle, and shows a tendency towards gradual growth. The disease incidence has increased markedly in the past four decades.

At present, the etiological classification criteria (1999) proposed by WHO Diabetes Experts Committee is commonly used as an international standard for diagnosing diabetes. The criteria are as follows: Type I diabetes melitus, with β cell damage, often leading to an absolute deficiency of insulin; Type II diabetes melitus, from inadequate insulin secretion and insulin resistance.

Most diabetic patients die of cardio-cerebrovascular and atherosclerosis disorders or diabetic nephropathy. As compared with the non-diabetic population, the mortality of diabetic population for all reasons increases by 1.5~2.7 times, the mortality for cardiovascular disease increases by 1.5~4.5 times, and lower limb skin ulcers and gangrene requiring amputation is 20 times higher.

As compared with the non-diabetic population, the prevalence of artery atherosclerosis among diabetic population is relatively high, the onset age is relatively young and disease progression is relatively fast. As an important component of metabolic syndrome, susceptible factors for known artery atherosclerosis such as obesity, hypertension, and lipid metabolic abnormality show a significant increase among the diabetic (mainlyT2 DM) population. Artery atherosclerosis mainly involves the aorta, coronary artery, cerebral artery, renal artery and limb peripheral artery, leading to coronary heart disease, ischemic or hemorrhagic cerebrovascular disease, renal atherosclerosis, limb atherosclerosis, etc.

At the cellular level, diabetes changes various cellular functions, including endothelial cells and smooth muscle cells, eventually resulting in vascular structure and function disorder.

Diabetes is the late manifestation of vascular lesions that result from hyperglycemia, with the mechanism as: mutual effect of gene polymorphism of eNOS and environmental factors, leading to endothelial function failure and nitric oxide synthesis reduction and thus resulting in vascular lesions. Much of the disorder is due to "advanced glycation end products" (AGES) as discussed earlier.

There is much evidence to suggest that by adding L-arginine to the diet of diabetic animals, it is possible to increase the synthesis of nitric oxide by endothelial NOS (NOS-3) in diabetic animals, so as to prevent the incidence of diabetic vascular lesions or improve the existing diabetic vascular lesions. Recently, other scholars have also discovered that exercise can increase NOS in the bodies of diabetic patients, thus prolonging the time before the vascular endothelium becomes injured. Such results have provided the basis for preventing and curing diabetic vascular endothelial injury by increasing the NO level in the bodies of patients.

Chapter Three
Helping Man to Avoid Cardio-cerebrovascular Diseases

Increasing nitric oxide to reduce cardiovascular diseases

Cardiovascular disease has the highest fatality rates in the world, presently greater than cancer. But with advancing age, cancer may become more prevalent. Over the last two decades, data on the incidence of cardiovascular diseases suggests an upward trend, especially for females. For females, the primary cause of death used to be cancer, but is now cardiovascular disease.

To a great extent, cardiovascular disease is a lifestyle disease, and can therefore be avoided by making changes to one's lifestyle. Unhealthy diets, such as saturated fat, red meat, hydrogenated oil added in packaged food, salt added in food, inadequate fruit and vegetable and inadequate intake of foodstuffs rich in antioxidants can all increase the risk of cardiovascular diseases. Furthermore, obesity and sitting for long periods of time without exercise further increase the incidence of cardiovascular diseases.

In 1998, three scientists were awarded with the Nobel Prize for discovering that nitric oxide is a signal molecule that spreads throughout the human body to protect it against cardiovascular disease and other diseases. Since nitric oxide can be promptly damaged by oxidants (saturated fat, inflammation, and oxygen free radicals relating to oxidative stress), it is extremely important for preventing nitric oxide deficiency to include foodstuffs rich in L-arginine and antioxidants in our diets.

While exercising, the skeleton and muscles are in continual motion, bringing nutrition to the peripheral tissues and cellular tissues and further accelerating the recovery of tissues. In the meanwhile, metabolism will also speed up. Therefore, when participating in sports and fitness activities, you will feel a pain in the legs and arms. However, it is necessary to exercise continuously. You will still feel a pain upon exercising for one week due to inadequate generation of nitric oxide. It is because of the above reason that physical exercise is very beneficial. Therefore, even light exercise can help us to increase the generation of nitric oxide. Nitric oxide not only can accelerate blood flow, but in the long term can also protect the cardiovascular system against the effects of diseases, due to the active action of the enzyme nitric oxide synthase (NOS) to produce NO Researchers have also discovered that, frequent exercise or repetition of one exercise also can regulate endothelial nitric oxide synthase. Genes can also be regulated so that the body will continue to generate nitric oxide. Therefore, in this way, more nitric oxide can be synthesized continuously. Exercise can also decrease free radicals leading to decreased oxidative stress, protecting the nitric oxide already formed in the human body and increasing content of nitric oxide in the body. Physical exercise can retard the speed of atherosclerosis, while nitric oxide can also reduce atherosclerosis and retard the speed of atherosclerosis considerably. Not only in terms of cardiovascular diseases, but also in central nervous system, nitric oxide can play an important role in neuronal transmission (i.e. memory).

Nitric oxide plays an important role in regulating vascular function and regulating the stability of blood pressure. Under a physiological state, when vessels are impacted by blood flow and perfusion pressure rises suddenly, as a messenger for balancing these effects, nitric oxide keeps blood flow through the organs relatively stable so that vessels are able to perform the function of self-regulation. Nitric oxide can lower the arterial blood pressure of the body as a whole, control the resting tension of different vascular beds throughout the body and increase blood flow as a major regulatory factor of blood pressure.

Relationship between nitric oxide and atherosclerosis and coronary heart disease

Atherosclerosis is also an inflammatory lesion of the artery, in addition to lipid accumulation, which may cause arterial walls to become thick and hard and lose elasticity and lumens to become narrow. Atherosclerosis is a vascular disease occurring as the human body ages. Generally, it first takes place during the teenage years and worsens during middle and old age. Its incidence is higher for males than females. In recent years, the disease has gradually increased in China and become one of the major causes for

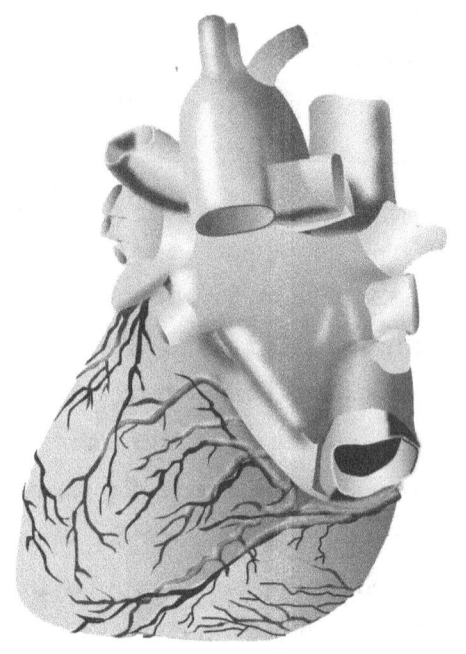

Structure of the heart (rear view)

death among the elderly. Previously women had less atherosclerosis perhaps due to their hormones, but with lifestyle changes their incidence of cardiovascular diseases is increasing.

Coronary artery heart disease (CHD), also known as coronary heart disease, is the most common form of heart disease. Its symptom expression is myocardial dysfunction or organic lesion due to coronary arterial stenosis and inadequate blood supply, and is therefore also known as ischemic heart disease (IHD). The main symptoms include a kind of squeezing pain generated in the center of the chest, which can shift to the neck, jaw, arm, rear back and stomach. Other possible symptoms include dizziness, short breath, sweating, shivering, and feeling faint. In severe cases, heart failure may cause death.

Due to the discovery of nitric oxide, the function of the endothelium and nitric oxide to maintain a healthy environment for vessels has been demonstrated. Nitric oxide regulates vascular tension and myocardial contractility, inhibits partial adhesion and aggregation of platelets and leukocyte adhesion inside vessels, inhibits the proliferation and migration of vascular smooth muscle cells, maintains the integrity of endothelial cells and thus inhibits the formation of thrombus. The main effects are as follows:

Nitric oxide has a relaxing effect. Nitric oxide released from vascular endothelial cells or neurons in the vessels can balance the vascular tension that results from the sympathetic nervous system and renin angiotension system. When nitric oxide binds to guanylate cyclase, the enzyme is activated so that guanosine triphosphate is converted into cGMP that again activates cGMP-dependent protein kinase to relax the vascular smooth muscles in the following ways: Intracellular Ca^{2+} decreases so that the smooth muscle is relaxed. Furthermore, nitric oxide can activate the potassium channels of cell membranes so that K^+ conductance increases, cells are hyperpolarized, voltage-dependent potassium channels are deactivated, intracellular Ca^{2+} decreases and smooth muscle is relaxed. These effects decrease the phosphorylation of the myosin filaments in smooth muscle to cause relaxation. Nitric oxide can prevent platelets from adhesion and aggregation on the vascular endothelium. When vascular endothelial cells are injured and collagen tissues of subintima are exposed in blood flow, platelets adhere and are partially aggregated, releasing such substances as serotonin and platelet-derived growth factor, which may promote the proliferation of smooth muscle cells and accelerate the incidence and development of atherosclerosis. Moreover, the nitric oxide released by vascular endothelial cells can inhibit the aggregation of platelets upon vascular injury, and prevent platelets from adhering to the vascular wall. Its mechanism is as follows: nitric oxide can increase cGMP in platelets, while the increased cGMP further causes a decrease of Ca^{2+} in platelets so as to inhibit their adhesion and aggregation.

Nitric oxide can also prevent leukocyte adhesion, thereby preventing the vascular endothelium from being damaged. Adhesion of leukocytes is the early contributing factor in the formation of a local inflammation and atherosclerosis. Since nitric oxide can affect the activity of cellular adhesive molecules or inhibit their expression so as to block leukocytes from adhering to vascular endothelium and maintain smooth blood flux, nitric oxide can prevent the formation of atherosclerosis.

Nitric oxide can inhibit the proliferation of vascular smooth muscle. It is now proven that nitric oxide is very likely to, through cGMP, be able to inhibit the mitosis of vascular smooth muscle cells, inhibit their proliferation and migration and thus reduce the generation of their collagen fiber and elastic fiber, thereby preventing the formation and development of artery atherosclerosis. As more and more experiments have indicated, nitric oxide shows a significant inhibiting effect in stimulating endothelial cells and decreases vascular smooth muscle cells and inflammation and atherogenesis.

Relationship between nitric oxide and cerebral thrombus

Cerebral thrombus is one of the ischemic cerebrovascular diseases and is most commonly observed among the middle-aged and elderly population, without any significant variation between the genders. It is caused by lesions to cerebrovascular walls. Generally, the onset of cerebral thrombus is relatively slow; it mostly takes dozens of hours or several days from onset to peak. The stroke may occur during sleep or while resting quietly. Some patients may have no presymptoms, but become hemiplegic or experience aphasia. But some other patients may experience its onset during the daytime often have presymptoms such as dizziness, limb numbness and asthenia and temporary cerebral ischemia. The most common cause of cerebral thrombus formation is atherosclerosis. The most common reason for brain thrombus is artery atherosclerosis. Brain artery atherosclerosis will cause roughening and narrowing of the inner part of the blood vessel. And in some conditions, e.g. decrease in blood pressure, restricted blood flow, increase in blood viscosity and platelet aggregation rate, blood coagulation factor will increase the formation rate of thrombus as well as to block blood flow and brain tissue support by this blood vessel through a lack of oxygen and nutrition, sometimes even resulting in death.

Just before cerebral thrombus is formed, cerebral blood flow slows down and eventually reaches stasis. After this, the body will exhibit different compensatory mechanisms. Other vascular endothelial cells with mild lesions accelerate synthesization to release nitric oxide and other vasodilators and anti-platelet agglutinating substances. With relatively strong organic compensatory function, it is described as a transient ischemia attack or TIA. When the body decompensates, adhesion and agglutination of platelets induce the formation of thrombus. The formation and early period of acute cerebral thrombus is associated with a drop in levels of nitric oxide; during the period of brain edema upon formation of thrombus, nitric oxide may be have a harmful effect on brain tissues. If nitric oxide donor treatment is administered in the early stages for patients exhibiting acute cerebral thrombus formation, the prognosis is likely to improve; in case of brain edema, it is better not to administer any nitric oxide donor treatment; instead antioxidant therapy should be considered.

Chapter Four
Diabetes Prevention and Treatment

Vascular lesions caused by diabetes are closely associated with a glucose metabolism disorder and common glycosylation of proteins (AGES), and lipid metabolism abnormality. At present, according to most specialists in the field, diabetic angiopathy is closely associated with endothelial dysfunction, and nitric oxide plays a very important role therein. The blood vessels of patients with diabetes, hypertension, tobacco use and probably obesity do not make enough nitric oxide.

Nitric oxide synthesis increases in suffering diabetes

Many scholars have noted that the capability of vascular endothelial cells of diabetic rats for synthesis of nitric oxide declines. Recent studies of cerebral arteries of diabetic rats demonstrated that diabetic rats showed more significant vasoconstriction due to pressure stimuli than the control rats did.

As some experiments have shown, in suffering from diabetes, aldose reductase activity increases, transforming increasing amounts of glucose into sorbitol, while generation of adenosine triphosphate (ATP) decreases and consumes more NADH II, resulting in a reduction in the synthesis of nitric oxide, which also requires NADH II. Scientists have also demonstrated that an aldose reductase inhibitor can cause the vasodilatation induced by acetylcholine of vessels of diabetic rats to return to normal.

Aminoguanidine (AG), a drug used for preventing and curing diabetic vascular complications, is also proven to have an effect in inhibiting aldose reductase activity, which can block glucose from transforming into sorbitol so that more NADH II will be used for the synthesis of nitric oxide, and may be one of the functional mechanisms of AG for preventing and curing diabetic vascular complications. While AG was found to decrease the formation of AGES in diabetics the clinical trials were terminated due to some toxic effects.

Nitric oxide activity declines in case of suffering diabetes

According to many scholars, for diabetic patients, nitric oxide synthesis of their vascular endothelium will not necessary decrease; during one stage or in one organ, its synthesis will instead increase, while deactivation of nitric oxide by some substances generated in patients suffering from diabetes is the main reason for nitric oxide-dependent vasodilatation failure.

In patients suffering from diabetes, vascular endothelium-dependent vasodilatation functional decline may be associated with the following factors: a decrease nitric oxide synthesis; an increase in nitric oxide deactivation; the process of nitric oxide diffusion from endothelium to smooth muscle is blocked; the function of some receptor changes (such as nitric oxide and guanylate cyclase receptor down-regulation); vasoconstrictive substances released by vascular endothelium increase, and the increased formation of reactive oxygen species to trap the nitric oxide formed.

Generation and development of diabetic angiopathy is not determined by one single factor, but as a result of the combined effect of multiple factors. At different stages of diabetes, the mechanism for different organs to hold a dominating position may differ. Recently, Watcher, et al have proposed that the change of nitric oxide in patients suffering from diabetes is a process that changes according to the disease's progress, i.e., nitric oxide compensatory synthesis increases in the early period and decreases in the late period.

As several studies have shown, by adding L-arginine to the diet of diabetic animals, it is possible to increase the synthesis of nitric oxide in diabetic animals, so as to prevent the incidence of diabetic vascular lesions or improve the existing diabetic vascular lesions. Recently, other scholars have also discovered that exercise can increase NOS in the body of diabetic patients, thus avoiding injury to the vascular endothelium. Such results have provided bases for preventing and curing diabetic vascular endothelial injury by increasing the NO level in bodies of patients.

However, diabetes like many other diseases, can be caused by multiple factors, which always makes treatment more complicated and challenging. However, nitric oxide seems to be a central factor if the vessels don't make enough.

Chapter Five
Nitric Oxide and Tumors

As a messenger, nitric oxide is involved in execution of various functions such as inflammatory response, signal delivery, vascular regulation and immune system regulation. Nitric oxide is broadly and intimately involved with the physiological functions and the clinical pathology of the digestive system, and has many functions including the development of gastrointestinal cancer. One might also be surprised to learn that the mood of an individual can also affect the production of nitric oxide synthase (NOS) in the body. For example laughing may increase nitric oxide formation. Therefore, if a person becomes sick, their mood may exacerbate their condition even further. In contrast, individuals in a good mood are more likely to release normally functioning enzymes continuously, thereby avoiding any inflammation within the body.

Nitric oxide and cancer

The role of nitric oxide in tumor growth and suppression is quite complex. Clearly many but not all tumors have increased levels of nitric oxide produced by inducible NOS (NOS-2). Also, high levels of nitric oxide can be toxic to bacteria, viruses, pathogens, normal cells and tumor cells, to prevent their growth. However, tumors are heterogeneous with a variety of cell types. Thus, biochemical studies often cannot determine if the increase of NOS-2 is in the tumor cells or other cells in and around the tumor. Laboratory studies are quite mixed with some suggesting that nitric oxide suppresses tumor growth and other studies do not support the concept. The final story is still out with regard to nitric oxide and cancer since many tumors have little or no nitric oxide receptors (i.e. soluble guanylate cyclase) for nitric oxide to have an effect. Obviously, much more research is required to answer these important questions that could then help develop some novel drug treatments for cancer prevention and tumor growth.

Dr Murad's laboratory is beginning to make some important progress answering these important questions.

Chapter Six
Activating the Brain

Scientists from Medical School of US Wake Forest University have published an article on Neuroscience network edition), stating that they have discovered that nitric oxide in the human body can help the human brain to "activate" in the morning so that we can process visual and aural information as well as other information from the senses as soon as we become conscious.

The first author of the article, Dr. Godwin (Assistant Professor of neurobiology and anatomy) stated: "we have obtained new knowledge about how our brain processes sense organ information. This will help us to develop a better understanding of problems observed in schizophrenia, attention deficit disorder and epilepsy."

By studying ferrets, scientists have begun to understand the important function of the nitric oxide molecule in maintaining human health. By slowing the decomposition of cyclic GMP in the penis, the drug Viagra increases blood flow. The medicine for heart disease,

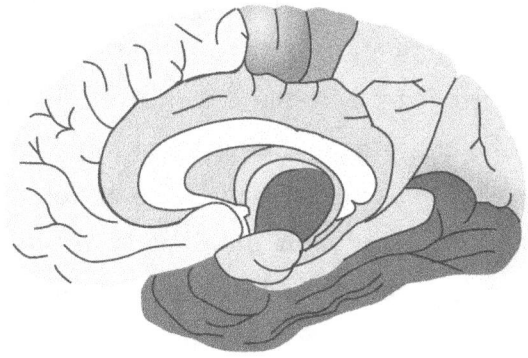

Facies medialis hemispherii cerebri

as discovered by Dr. Murad, nitroglycerine, is transformed by the body into nitric oxide to broaden the diameter of blood vessels and reduce angina pectoris. In the brain, the brain stem will naturally release a small amount of NO to the thalamus area during daytime, but scientists have little knowledge of its use. Nitric oxide is released in a state of awakening or brain arousal. By conducting a motion study, Godwin and his colleagues discovered that an increase of nitric oxide shows a surprising effect on sense organ information from eye to brain. Godwin said: "just like a computer that needs to start the operating system before processing complex applications, nitric oxide is released when the brain awakes and lays a foundation for complex brain operation by enhancing the processing of early information." The sense organ information from eyes, skin and ears first reaches the thalamus. The thalamus plays the role of access control, which either allows information to reach the cortex in control of thinking or prevents information from passing through. Scientists know that the thalamus will send information to the cerebral cortex, but were previously unclear about the effect of nitric oxide on information feedback from the cortex. Godwin said: "we discovered that nitric oxide released to thalamus enhances the communication between thalamus and cortex. This represents a brand-new insight into cerebral communication." According to his explanation, the visual information received by the cortex from the thalamus is just a small part of the entire image, equivalent to just one long line of pixels compared with a digital image. The cortex then establishes a complex method of expression and feeds back information to the thalamus for selecting the information required for completion of the image. Nitric oxide then enhances the feedback process. During the research, the scientists isolated the input information of the thalamus into two groups: one is input from eyes and the other is the feedback input from the cortex. Originally, they expected to discover that nitric oxide could enhance the signal from eyes, but on the contrary, they found that nitric oxide weakened the signal of eyes and enhanced, instead, the feedback signal from the cortex. It seems that such small molecule can allow the cortex to control information traffic from the thalamus to a degree previously unimaginable. Though it has not yet been proven, it is possible that other sense organs may also operate in the same way. These results show the way the brain communicates with itself. Moreover, it appears that different parts of the brain are more cooperative and flexible than previously imagined. Generally, it is thought that visual signals are transmitted directly from the eye to the cortex, but it is now clear that visual and other sense organ information is managed in a similar fashion to information in a computer circuit, in that each part's intensity will rise and fall in accordance with each of the brain's various states of consciousness.

Clearly, it has been known for some years that various neurons in the brain produce and release nitric oxide, but the extent of this network and the functions are only partially known.

Chapter Seven
Improvement of Alzheimer's Disease

Recently, neuroscientists have begun to pay more attention to the role of nitric oxide in neural conduction: no matter whether nerve synapses are connected or not, nitric oxide can promote communication between neurons. As experimental results show, inducing the inhibiting cerebral capacity of nitric oxide will affect the cerebral capacity of long-term memory.

Other cerebral researchers have begun to test the role nitric oxide plays in diseases such as Alzheimer's disease (senile dementia) and Parkinson's disease. From the bodies of patients suffering from such diseases, they discovered the circumstances under which a sharp decrease of nitric oxide yield can be observed in the brains of patients suffering from these diseases.

As various data provided in reports from Nature magazine show, reductions of nitric oxide yield may hinder the storage of memory and reduce cerebral blood flow. In turn, decrease of cerebral blood flow may immediately produce a kind of plaque known as beta amyloid, which increase and accumulates in vessels, as is the case in bodies of patients of several cerebral degenerative diseases including senile dementia. The chemical nature of such plaques is different from that of the atherosclerosis plaques that block cardiac arteries. However, Beta amyloidal plaques will also damage the endothelial cells of smaller cerebral vessels. Nitric oxide is such an important and omnipresent substance in the human body that leading scholars in this field have begun to draw attention to its crucial role in the human health and the numerous biological functions that it performs. Indeed, some diseases that might at first seem unrelated, such as senile dementia, diabetes and hemorrhoids, all have one point in common: all of these diseases are either caused or intensified by nitric oxide.

Chapter Eight
Improvement of Sleep Quality

Sleeping is one of the most familiar activities in our daily lives; humans spend about 1/3 of their lives asleep. In a sleeping state, we can rest our brain and body, allowing each to relax and recover. Sleeping is helpful for our daily work and study, and improvements of sleeping quality assure a corresponding increase in the quality of our daily work, study and life.

Insomnia, or lack of sleep, can be classified into 3 types: sleeping difficulties in the early stages of sleep, which is the most common form of insomnia; Interrupted sleep during the night; waking excessively early and failing to fall sleep again in the later stages of sleep. Individuals suffering from insomnia are less likely to experience paradoxical sleep, which can easily induce arousal

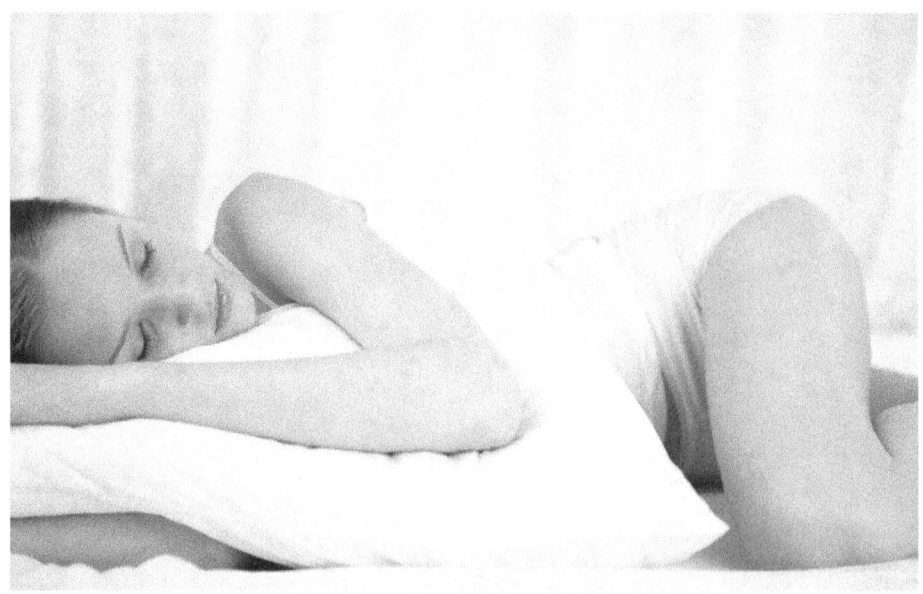

Improvement of sleep

response from brain waves.

Nitric oxide influences the biological factors that promote sleep in several ways. Current research on incurring and regulatory mechanism of sleeping are conducted with a focus on sleeping factors, according to which endogenous sleeping induced-matter and sleeping inhibited-matter form a complex regulatory network system that acts on the neural structure for sleeping-waking rhythm control. Studies prove that in the human body, sleep is influenced by several factors, including interleukin-1, tumor necrosis factor (TNF), growth hormone releasing hormone, vasoactive peptide, prostaglandin and classical neurotransmitter, 5-HT.

Additionally, substances such as acetylcholine, norepinephrine and dopamine, all of which play an important role in regulating sleep patterns, are generally called sleeping factors. At present, research indicates that many sleeping factors can promote the production of nitric oxide. According to some scholars, as a messenger molecule, nitric oxide produced in waking leads to a series of chain responses and results in the production and aggregation of sleep-promoting factors. Since nitric oxide has a very short half life, the central nervous system continues to produce nitric oxide, for continual production of sleeping factors.

Chapter Nine
Potentiation of Learning Memory

Classification by duration is the most basic and widely accepted classification of memory. Focusing on duration, memory can be classified into 3 different types: sensory memory, short-term memory and long-term memory.

The term short-term memory model has been replaced by the concept of "working memory" over the last 25 years, and can be divided into 3 systems: short-term visual impressions formed by spatial vision; voice information stored within the voice circuit, which can remain stored for long periods through continual repetition; the central execution system which manages the above two systems and associates information with the establishment of long term memory content. Long-term memory content is organized and managed not only by subject, but also by time. A new experience or a motion model obtained upon practicing will first go to working memory for short- term recording, where information can be read quickly, but in a limited capacity. For economic reasons, this information must eventually be deleted. Important information or information linked with other information through an "association" effect will be transmitted to the medium and long-term memory, while unimportant information will be deleted. Some scientists believe that memory capacity is limited and that some unwanted memory is deleted in order to store new memory. Other scientists believe that the brain's capacity for memory is unlimited and with considerable capacity to store information.

When memory content is more frequently read, or one motion is frequently repeated, the feedback will be more precise, evaluation of this content shall be prioritized, and the process will be optimized. The latter point means that unimportant information will be deleted or stored in another place. Memory capacity is related to the number of connections between various kinds of content, as well an evaluation of the emotional importance of this information.

Nitric oxide has multiple effects in the central nervous system. As a messenger, it is involved in the process of hippocampal long-term potentiation (LTP) and cerebellar long-term depression (LTD). Hippocampla LTP is a memory model occurring in synapses, which is considered to be the cellular base for learning memory. In the course of LTP formation, after glutamate activates the NMD receptor passage, calcium enters into the postsyaptic membrane and activates nitric oxide synthase; the nitric oxide generated diffuses from the postsynapse to the presynapse to react with guanylate cyclase or adenosine diphosphate-ribose transferase (ADPRT), and the activated ADPRT can cause the acylation of other ADP-glucose, so that ion passage activity changes, or sensitivity of the release process of neurotransmitter to calcium increases, thus resulting in the increasing release of presynapse neurotransmission, presynapse conduction and formation of learning memory.

Chapter Ten
Regulation of Visual System

Ocular structure

The eyeball wall is principally composed of three layers: outer, middle and inner. The outer layer consists of the cornea and sclera. The first 1/6 is transparent cornea, while the remaining 5/6 is white sclera, commonly known as "eye white". The outer layer plays the role of maintaining the shape of eyeball and protecting intraocular tissues. The cornea is the main channel for light to enter the eyes and form an image. It also as plays a role in protecting the eyes and is of great importance to human perception. Sclera consists of a compacted collagen fiber structure and is consequently non-transparent, milk white and firm in quality. The middle layer, also known as uveal and uvea, is composed of rich pigments and vessels, which may be divided into three parts: The iris is ring-shaped and is located at the front of the eye and before the lens. Other properties of the iris include radial wrinkles, collectively called texture, and uneven recess on the surface.

The color of the iris varies from person to person, and is decided by the genetic make-up of the individual. In the center is one 2.5~4mm circular hole, called the pupil. The ciliary is connected to the root of the iris in front and to the choroid in the rear. The sclera can be found to its exterior, while its interior is connected to the lens via suspensory ligaments. The choroid is located between the sclera and retina. The blood circulation of the choroid provides nutrition to the ectoretina, and its rich pigments play a role of a "darkroom". The inner layer consists of the retina, which is one layer of transparent membrane. This area is the first where neural information is delivered to allow the formation of vision. It is a fine network structure with metabolic and physiological functions. At the end opposite to the optical axis of the retina is the macular central fovea. The macular area is a special area on the retina that is visually most sensitive, with a diameter of about 1~3mm; in the center is a small foveola, i.e., central fovea. At about

3mm to the side of macular area near the nose is a faint red area with a diameter of about 1.5mm, known as the optic disc, or the optic nerve head. The optic disc is where ganglion cell axons exit the eye to form the optic nerve. There are no light sensitive rods or cones to respond to a light at this point. This causes a break in the visual field called "the blind spot" or the "physiological blind spot".

The intraocular compartment and restricted substance: the intraocular compartment includes anterior chamber, posterior chamber and vitreous cavity. Restricted substances include the aqueous humor, crystalline lens and vitreum. All three are transparent, and collectively called, together with cornea, the dioptric media. The aqueous humor is produced by the ciliary process in the anterior chamber, and has the effect of nourishing the cornea, crystalline lens and vitreum while maintaining intraocular pressure (IOP). The crystalline lens is a hyaline body rich in elastic tissue, the shape of a biconvex lens, and located behind the iris and pupil and before the vitreum. The vitreum is a transparent plastic mass, filling up 4/5 of the post-eyeball cavity. Its main content is water. The vitreum has a refractive effect, and also plays the role of supporting the retina.

Optic nerve and visual pathway: the optic nerve is part of the central nervous system. The visual information obtained by the retina is delivered, via the visual nerve, to the brain. The visual pathway is the path from the point where the retina receives visual information to the cerebral optic cortex. The entire nerve impulse transmission of vision is conducted along this path.

Accessory organs of the eye include the eyelid, conjunctiva, lacrimal apparatus, ophthalmic rectus muscles, orbital fat body and orbital fasciae.

Effects of nitric oxide on eyes

1) Effect of nitric oxide on ocular circulation

In the eye nitric oxide can be produced by the choroidal, vascular endothelial cells in the retina, the retinal rod cell outer segment, the retinal nerve element, choroidal vascular bypass nerve fiber, and retinal pigment epithelia cells. Clearly, nitric oxide also has the effect of regulating ocular circulation. It can also regulate fluid turnover and removal in the eye by affecting the ciliary body and anterior chamber blood flow.

According to the latest research, the independent regulation of retinal vessels may be controlled by the following two mechanisms: one uses nitric oxide released by retinal endothelial cells in blood circulation; the other uses nitric oxide released by choroid ganglion plexus. Nitric oxide produced from retinal vessels can cause arterioles to respond quickly to changes in blood pressure and oxygenation, while choroidal segment cells may play an important role in regulating the rapid dilatation response of choroidal vessels. Since nitric oxide can easily pass through cell membranes and intercellular space, nitric oxide produced by the choroid can diffuse into retinal arterioles in order to regulate their contraction. Many studies have shown that by dilating vessels and increasing blood flow, nitric oxide can play a role in regulating the central nervous system and blood flow throughout arteries both in and outside eyeball and retinal capillary. By regulating blood circulation, such symptoms as ocular fatigue and visual impairment due to long-term use of the eye can be improved.

2) Effects of nitric oxide on age-related macular degeneration

Age-related macular degeneration (AMD) is a common geriatric disease, with 20 million patients in USA alone. In China, more than 50 million patients suffer from this disease, showing a distinct upward trend. For more than 2/3 of AMD patients, the main cause for choroidal neovascularization is the early choroidal circulation failure. To prevent this condition, it is necessary to improve and promote choroidal blood flow. Endothelial nitric oxide synthase is observable in optic choroidal vascular endothelial cells and by regulating the release of nitric oxide, vasodilatation and blood flow functions to regulate the choroid. In up-regulating protein expression and enzyme activity of endothelial nitric oxide synthase in endothelial cells, the amount of nitric oxide released is increased to promote choroidal blood flow, thus facilitating the prevention and cure of degenerative macular eye disease.

3) Effect of nitric oxide on the optic nervous system

The eye is the most important of the human sensory organs. About 80% of knowledge and memory in the brain is captured using the eye. The eye can identify different colors and light before changing these visual images into neural signals to be transmitted to the brain. As a new neurotransmitter, nitric oxide is widely distributed in the tertiary neurons of the visual system. Under normal biological conditions, together with some neurotransmitters and neuropeptide, nitric oxide is involved in optic development and integration and delivery of visual information and is associated with the hippocampal LTP effect. Nitric oxide is involved in the synaptic plasticity of the visual nervous system, indicating that nitric oxide may play an important role in the pathogenesis of deprived amblyopia.

Chapter Eleven
Protection of Liver and Lungs

Protection of liver and lungs

It is widely known that excessive smoking and alcohol consumption have adverse effects on our health. Smoking too much will cause emphysema and lung cancer. Excessive drinking will damage the liver. Fatigue due to a lack of sleep and exhaustion will also harm the health of the liver and kidneys. Additionally, additives in food, pesticide residues in vegetables and rotten food exert a heavy burden to kidney, liver and stomach. Let us first look at the effects of smoking. Upon

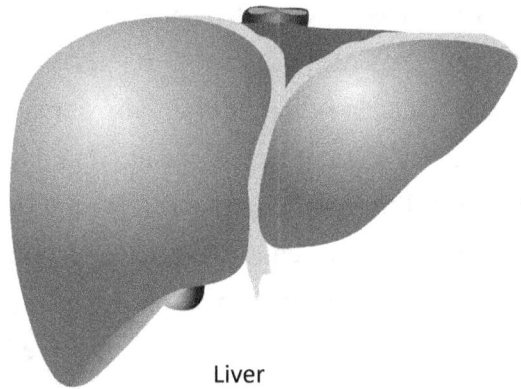

Liver

being inhaled into the lungs, smoking will form tobacco residue inside. As tobacco residue attaches itself to the inside lung, large amounts of tars and inflammation will be produced. According to the research, one cigarette can produce 30 million reactive oxygen species (ROS). Therefore, the more cigarettes smoked, the more ROS will be produced, causing oxidative damage to pulmonary tissue, which is closely associated with the formation of emphysema and cancer cell lesions. As data shows, it is necessary to take Vitamin C equal to 20~30 oranges to resist the bad oxygen produced by smoking one cigarette. It therefore goes without saying that smoking causes great harm to the human body as it can injure many other tissues as well. Next is alcohol consumption; once too much alcohol is consumed, it must be detoxified in the liver, where alcohol is oxidized to acetaldehyde before being decomposed into acetic acid. During the course of decomposition, a large amount of ROS will be produced in order for the oxidation of alcohol to take place, damaging hepatic cells and leading to alcoholic hepatitis in the process. Additionally, chemical additives in food also cause severe harm. According to available statistics, food additives are microscopic, but we take in at least 50 types of food additives on average every day. For such substances, toxins must be excreted by the kidney and metabolized partially in the liver, thus allowing ROS to penetrate cells. Over a long period, this will cause a severe burden and damage to organs.

The main effects and biological processes attributable to nitric oxide that take place in the lung include the following: As an important vasodilator in the body, it can catalyze the generation of cGMP for dilating vascular smooth muscle; acetylcholine, bradykinin and other vasodilators all dilate vessels through the mediation of nitric oxide, exhibiting an important effect in maintaining pulmonary vasodilatation; as the only non-cholinergic and non-adrenergic neurotransmitter of the respiratory system, it relaxes airway smooth muscle and dilates the airway; it plays an important role in host defense; when a phagocyte is activated by endotoxin or T-cells, a massive amount of nitric oxide and other inflammatory media are produced to kill germs and tumor cells; it promotes the dissolution of fibrous protein, inhibits the aggregation of platelets; it inhibits the aggregation of neutrophil, reduces the expression of adhesion molecule, and has an anti-inflammatory effect; it mediates inflammatory apoptosis and production of pro- inflammatory cytokines, as well as regulating the direction of the inflammatory response. Moderate amounts of nitric oxide therefore have an important protecting function in the human body.

By dilating pulmonary vessels, endogenous nitric oxide plays an important role in regulating the physiological and pathological process of pulmonary circulation. Therefore, exogenous inhalation of nitric oxide is crucial importance to the treatment of different types of pulmonary hypertension. Since nitric oxide can be combined with hemoglobin in the blood stream for quick deactivation, inhalation of nitric oxide only acts on pulmonary vessels, without any effects on the systemic circulation. Clinical studies have also proven that inhalation of low-density (20~40ppm) nitric oxide can significantly reduce primary pulmonary hypertension, congenital cardiopathy and pulmonary hypertension in people with a normal physiological status due to hypoxia. Thus, inhaling very low concentrations of nitric oxide are very helpful in premature blue babies with pulmonary hypertension due to incomplete lung development and constricted pulmonary vessels.

By regulating hepatic blood flow, nitric oxide affects the oxygenation of hepatic tissues. When nitric oxide synthesis is depressed, hepatic sinusoidal blood flow decreases, platelets aggregate, micro thrombus is formed and leukocytes adhere, aggravating the effect of oxidative damage to hepatic tissues. However, when nitric oxide synthesis increases, it can improve tissue ischemia, and reduce the effect of oxidative damage.

Chapter Twelve
Improvement of Enterogastric Functions

Digestion and absorption are important functions that allow the human body to acquire energy and survive. After the complex process of digestion and decomposition in the gastrointestinal tract, food, including vitamins, metal salts and trace elements, are broken down into small molecular substances and absorbed by the intestinal tract and become, after hepatic processing, the substances necessary for the human body for use in the systemic tissues. Meanwhile the leftover substances that are not absorbed and have no nutritional value are excreted as feces. In addition, the digestive system also has the capacity to remove certain toxic substances and pathogenic microorganisms. The digestive system also secretes various hormones that regulate various systemic physiological functions.

Completion of digestion depends on the physical (motion) effect and chemical (secretion) effects of the digestive tract. These two processes are coordinated through regulation by nerves, enzyme secretion by the stomach, intestine and pancreas and various hormone factors and body fluids.

Digestive system diseases include diseases of organs such as the esophagus, stomach, intestine, liver, bile, pancreas, peritoneum, mesentery and omentum. Digestive system diseases are among the most common. In China, deaths related to gastric cancer and liver cancer rank the second and third respectively among the most common malignant tumor-related deaths, and there has been a rising trend in the prevalence of colorectal and pancreatic cancer in recent years as well. Digestive ulcers are one of the most common digestive diseases.

Under normal physiological conditions, the gastroduodenal mucosa is often in contact with strongly erosive gastric acids. When activated in an acidic environment it can hydrolyze protein. In addition, it is often invaded by various harmful substances ingested by the body, but can resist the damage of most invasive elements and maintain the integrity of the mucosa using a series of defending and repairing mechanisms. The eventual formation of digestive ulcers is due to the digestion of mucosa by gastric acid/pepsin. As pepsin activity is pH-dependent and is lost when pH>4, consideration is mainly given to gastric acid when discussing the pathogenesis and treatment measures of digestive ulcers. The fact that without acid, ulcers are rare and drugs inhibiting gastric acid secretion can promote recovery from ulcers has proven that gastric acid has a decisive effect on the formation of ulcers. The harmful effects of gastric acid are observable only when the normal mucosa defending and repairing function is damaged. In addition the bacterium Helicobacter Pylori can reside in the stomach and through unknown mechanisms can increase the development of gastro-duodenal peptic ulcers.

Nitric oxide synthase (NOS) is distributed throughout human digestive tract tissues, with different quantities in different areas. It is mostly found in the small intestine, as well as in different layers of the gastrointestinal wall. Nitric oxide is involved with the regulation of gastrointestinal mucosa blood flow, the regulation of the gastric mucosa secretion function, the immune protective barrier of the gastrointestinal mucosa, and the regulation of gastrointestinal motility. It performs an important repairing function in the event of any mucosa injury.

The integrity of the gastrointestinal tract mucosa relies on the balance between the different protective factors and damaging elements to which the mucosa is exposed, while protective factors in the mucosa include the regulation of mucosa blood flow, continual secretion of alkaline mucus and the proliferation and recovery of mucosa epithelium. The turnover of the intestinal mucosa cells is one of the most rapid in the body with cells replaced every few days.

Nitric oxide plays an important role in regulating blood flow in the gastric mucosa and maintaining the integrity of the mucosa. Nitric oxide can regulate the basic tension of gastric mucosa vessels, and increase blood flow. As for mucosa damage resulting from ischemia-reperfusion due to stress and excessive drinking, nitric oxide can reduce the damage through the following mechanisms: dilating vessels, improving blood supply to tissue, inhibiting platelets adhesion to the vascular endothelium, and eliminating ROS. Nitric oxide is also of considerable importance to the processes that regulate gastric mucosa secretion. It can also cause an increase in the concentration of the epithelial cell cGMP found in the gastric mucosa, as well as an increase of mucus secretion, and a significant reduction of gastric acid secretion.

Nitric oxide can improve intestinal injury due to the platelet activation factor, and has the effect of resisting shock and protecting the endothelium in the ischemia-reperfusion model. It also has the effect of a chemical barrier to adhesion and exudation of leukocytes, as well as promoting the repair of epithelium after acute injury. It can also cause relaxation of the intestine in its peristaltic movements.

As an important non-epinephrine and non-cholinergic nerve depressive neurotransmitter inside the gastrointestinal tract, nitric oxide plays an important role in regulating the gastrointestinal tract. The immune function of nitric oxide also plays a role in the gastrointestinal tract. Formation of nitric oxide may be the first line of defense in the body for cells to resist foreign pathogens as well as being a mediator for immune signals. Despite the knowledge about nitric oxide since the discovery of Dr. Murad in 1977, much remains still unknown and requires more research.

Chapter Thirteen
Potentiation of Sexual Function

Studies have shown, individuals of advanced years in the region of South Xinjiang still can maintain an active sexual life on a weekly basis. How is sexual capability related to lifespan? In fact, each time cells are about to divide, it is necessary to first carry out gene duplication, while the chromosome genomes in the cell's nucleus change from one to two. The scientific name for the two ends of a chromosome is telosome. Telomerase is an enzyme that influences the repair of the chromosome ends and has higher enzyme activity in human germ cells. Increase of telomerase assures the duplication of genes, activates cells, and thus delays aging by repairing the chromosomes.

Late 1980s Massachusetts statistics for 40 to 70 year-old males show that 52% suffer from erectile dysfunction, (mild 17.2%, moderate 25.2%, severe 9.6%). In mitochondria, scientists have discovered the significance of nitric oxide synthase (NOS) toward human sexual capability and longevity. Without any hormones, it has no toxic side effects on the human body and can help people to maintain a state of vigorous health well into old age. As many of men aged 70~80 indicated, upon supplementing nitric oxide, sexual capability was enhanced to various extents. This is because germ cells become active after supplementing nitric oxide, following which sexual capability and sexual desire increased accordingly. Nitric oxide also increases penile erection as discussed below.

Nitric oxide is a small molecular substance for starting penile erection

More than 20 years ago, scientists determined through their research that nitric oxide was the key molecular substance necessary for penile erection. Sexual stimuli around the penis stimulates nerve endings to release nitric oxide, thus relaxing the vascular smooth muscle of the penis (which are in contraction in their normal state). Blood enters by perfusion and dilates the vessels of the corpus carvernosum tissues, so that it erects with increased blood flow like a balloon charged with gas. However, it was not clear for a long time how penile erection was maintained.

On March 19, 2005, the National Academy of Sciences (PNAS) published a research report by Arthur Bernett (urinary physiologist of Johns Hopkins University, Maryland, USA), et al, which indicated that nitric oxide might play an important role in maintaining penile erection. Just as a rod and ropes might support a circus tent, something must be used to maintain penile erection. According to Bernett, et al, nitric oxide may play a role in maintaining penile erection. They carefully observed and studied NOS, the enzyme discovered in penile vascular endothelial cells and corpus carvernosum tissues responsible for the production of nitric oxide. They used rats for experiments, applying mild current stimulation to their penis for 15sec and consequently found that it could increase the production of their active NOS by 40%. In turn, chemical substances inhibiting the enzyme NOS could reduce the blood pressure inside of the penis, indicating that this enzyme is necessary for maintaining erection.

Yet Bernett, et al also noted that NOS appeared to play a role in maintaining penile erection, as the penis did not remain in erection without the presence of endothelial NOS in the experiment; no such problem occurred if only neural NOS (NOS-1) was missing. Bernett, et al concluded that neural NOS initiated the initial erection of penis, which is then maintained by endothelial NOS (NOS-3).

According to Burnett, since female genitals also contain endothelial NOS, the research result is effective as a treatment for both male and female sexual dysfunction. According to Tom Ryge, a urinary expert from California University, the research has led to the development of a new concept to use in the study of the many diseases that affect endothelial cells. For instance high cholesterol may disturb NOS, and thus cause male impotence.

Chapter Fourteen
Prolonging of Female's Reproductive Ability

The prospect of uncovering the key to male impotence was no doubt exciting for Bernett and his team. However, not wanting to appear biased in their research, they decided to focus on the effect of NOS on female sexual function performance as well. This decision would lead to new insights as illuminating as their previous male-oriented research.

The problem Bernett, et al encountered was that it was hard to find individuals willing to participate in experiments concerning the biological mechanisms of the clitoris. Fortunately, they were able to find 4 patients who wished to undergo male to female trans-gender plastic surgery. Bernett and his colleagues made requests to these individuals that they participate in experiments to advance our understanding of a crucial field in medicine. Luckily the 4 patients and their guardians were sufficiently open-minded and happily agreed to cooperate.

Each of the 4 patients is atypical in their biological gender identity.

3 of them were female pseudohermaphrodites, owing to congenital adrenal proliferation, and were aged 2 months, 3 years and 12 years respectively; another female aged 17 was a true hermaphrodite.

Since being diagnosed with gender differentiation abnormality, these patients had been in medical therapy. During plastic surgery, they all exhibited production of normal female sex hormones. The testing items obtained during the course of plastic surgery of feminine genital included the glans clitoris and corpora cavernosa clitoris. To ensure the study as more complete and accurate, Bernett et al also obtained more integral pudendal tissues from one 46-year-old deceased normal female within 12 hours in addition to the 4 patients. Her pelvic anatomy was complete, without being injured due to disease or cause of death.

As the thesis published on Journal of Urology (1997) showed, by using the technique of immunohisotochemistry, Bernett et al discovered that NOS can be observed in the human clitoris, the corpora cavernosa clitoris has more neuron nitric oxide synthase (nNOS or NOS-1) than the glans clitoris, while the glans clitoris contains a comparatively large amount of endothelial nitric oxide synthase (eNOS or NOS-3). This discovery showed that in this respect, the biological properties of the female genital organs correlate strongly to those of the male anatomy: the main explanation for hyperemia and erection of the male corpus cavernosum is the nitric oxide produced by nNOS (NOS-1).

NOS-1 is distributed in parts of the nervous system, and the nitric oxide synthesized can regulate nerves and transmit signals, such as those involved in various physiological processes including learning and memory. It also has the effect in regulating cerebral blood flow and in some peripheral nervous systems, it plays a role as a neurotransmitter, with the function of controlling such organs such as the intestine and stomach. According to some studies, the development of some neurodegenerative diseases is associated with nitric oxide; and nitric oxide deficiency will lead to senile dementia, among other conditions.

Additionally some American scientists have recently discovered through their research that nitric oxide can help males to recover the erection function and increase blood flow and can also help females to improve their sexual functions.

116

According to researchers, the ova excreted from the ovary by females of advanced ages are also subject to the aging process. The time for such ova to become fertilized for conception is usually shorter than that for the ova of young females. For this reason, it is usually hard for elderly females to conceive.

During this research, researchers studied 1,500 newly excreted white-rat ova. The results of the study showed that the ova that failed to combine with sperm immediately started to age. By the 6th hour, such ova were basically incapable of undergoing fertilization. After this time period, if sperm was implanted, there was a significantly higher probability of fetus malformation.

During this period, using varying dosages of nitric oxide, the researchers treated the white-rat ova. It was observed that nitric oxide can delay the aging process of white-rat ova as well as the increase in the release of molecules designed to stop fertilization. The researchers also discovered that ova treated with nitric oxide can delay other aging processes that affect fertilization.

According to the researchers, their research results indicated that nitric oxide can not only be used to prolong the time window for elderly females to conceive, but also can be used to promote the fertilization of IVF ova. Additionally, the research also discovered that nitric oxide may be used to help prevent the fetus from experiencing a genetic mutation during the early stages of development and can be used to prevent problems common among elder females, such as frequent miscarriages.

Chapter Fifteen
Right of Life and Death for Cells

The immune functions of leukocytes are performed in part through the application of their adhesion abilities, and the adhesive effect of leukocytes is mediated by various adhesion molecules. In a normal physiological state, leukocytes should not adhere to the vascular wall. To prevent this, nitric oxide secreted by basal endothelial cells diffuses into leukocytes, and, mediating the increase of cGMP, causes leukocytes to remain stable in blood and nonadhesive. In experiments where rats were injected with NOS inhibitors (to reduce nitric oxide), it was demonstrated that it is possible to increase the adhesion ability of leukocytes with the vascular wall by 10 times after injecting arginine. It is also possible to cause endothelial cells to secrete nitric oxide, stop leukocytes from adhering to and infiltrating the vascular intima, relieve the ischemia of experimented animals' myocardium and reperfusion injury, and reduce infarcted myocardial area. According to research by scientists from Duke University Medical Center, nitric oxide displays a critical effect in the life and death of human cells and even controls the "right" of each cell to live or die. Nitric oxide molecules are present everywhere in the human body. The researchers at Duke University discovered that nitric oxide molecule shows a "convening" effect on protein networks that guides the most basic activities of cells, and such proteins can often decide the life or death of cells.

On the basis of this new discovery, we have achieved an even greater understanding of the effect of the nitric oxide molecule on human cells. With these new insights, scientists expect to find out the cause for such diseases related to cellular decay such as heart failure, asthma, and Alzheimer's disease.

As other studies show, nitric oxide has a direct relationship with the functions of immune cells. Immune cells release a considerable amount of nitric oxide in order to sterilize and prevent virus and parasitic infection. Nitric oxide is involved in the production of marrow cells and it has been demonstrated that increased "killer T cells" in the immune system occur due to nitric oxide.

As research results show, nitric oxide can be produced in various cells of the human body. When in vivo internal toxin or T cells activate phagocytes and polymorphonuclear leukocytes, a huge amount of inducible nitric oxide synthase and superoxide anion free radicals can be produced in order to synthesize a huge amount of nitric oxide and hydrogen peroxide and superoxide (ROS), which play an extremely important role in killing invasive bacteria, fungi and other microbes and tumor cells, organic foreign matters, as well as in the repair of inflammation related injury.

It is now thought that nitric oxide released by the activated phagocyte may have an influence on the extermination of target cells in ways such as the inhibition of the TCA cycle in the mitochondria of target cells, and deoxyribonucleic acid (DNA) synthesis of cells. Nitric oxide resulting from an immune response mechanism also shows a toxic effect on adjacent tissues and cells that can produce nitric oxide synthase. Some tissue injuries in association with the immune system and abnormal dilatation and permeability of vessels may all be partially associated with the presence of nitric oxide. For example, with serious infections and sepsis the toxins and inflammatory cytokines released markedly increase nitric oxide formation to kill the pathogen, but the blood vessels also dilate excessively and cause blood pressure to decrease and to cause "septic shock".

Chapter Sixteen
Assistance in Improving Immunity and Playing Anti-fatigue Effect

Nitric oxide helps to improve immunity

Immune functions include the specific immune function and non-specific immune function.

So-called specific immunity refers to the process by which lymphocytes produce relevant antibodies that target one specific antigen or carry out partial cellular response in order to complex or kill specific antigens. According to the difference of their incidence and function, lymphocytes in blood can be classified into two types: T lymphocytes and B lymphocytes. Cellular immunity is mediated mainly through T cells that account for 80%~90% of the total volume of lymphocytes in the blood. After T cells become sensitized cells when stimulated by antigens, their effect is manifested in three ways: they directly contact and attack foreign matter with specific antigenicity, such as tumor cells and allograft cells, they secrete various lymphokines, and they damage the cells containing pathogens and inhibit virus proliferation. B cells and T cells have a mutual effect on each other and enhance each other to kill pathogenic microbes. Humoral immunity is actualized mainly through B cells. Upon becoming plasma cells with immune activity due to antigen stimulation, such cells produce and secrete various antibodies, as well as immunoglobulin for different antigens. B cells include rich rough endoplasmic reticulum, with flourishing protein synthesis. Through immune reactions with relevant antigens, antibodies can neutralize, aggregate or dissolve antigens, to eliminate their harmful effects.

Like specific immunity, non-specific immunity, also known as natural immunity or inherent immunity, is a genetic characteristic acquired by human beings through a long period of evolution. For this reason, people are born with non-specific immunity capabilities. The non-specific immune system includes: tissue barriers (the skin and mucosa system, blood-brain barrier, placental barrier, etc); inherent immune cells (phagocytic cell, killer cells, dendritic cells, etc); inherent immune molecules (complement, cytokine, enzyme substances, etc). However, specific immunity is acquired through a process. For instance, swine flu spreads rapidly among pigs, but is not concerned with human beings. This is because by nature, man will not suffer such diseases, as inflammatory response is also an ability man is born with. Inherent immunity can promptly respond to different types of invading pathogenic microbes and play an important role in the start-up and effects of specific immunity processes.

The immune system is responsible for three major functions: Physiological defense: the human body resists the invasion of pathogens and their toxic products to prevent the onset of any infectious diseases. Self-stabilization: human tissue cells metabolize continuously, with new cells constantly replacing aging and injured cells. The immune system can quickly identify aging and dead cells and remove them from the body in order to keep the human body stable. Immune surveillance: the immune system performs the function of identifying, killing and removing in vivo mutant cells, thereby preventing the incidence of tumors. These functions are known collectively as immune surveillance. Immune surveillance is one of the most basic functions of the immune system.

Nitric oxide is a component of the in vivo non-specific defense response system. Being stimulated by in vivo phagocytes, neutrophils and other cytokines and the bacterial endotoxin lipopolysaccharide or endotoxin, it may initiate nitric oxide synthase to begin synthesizing large amounts of nitric oxide. One of the effects of nitric oxide is to kill bacteria, fungi, parasites and tumor cells. It also displays a toxic effect on in vivo tumor cells, but while providing the immune effect, it also has a toxic effect on those cells manifesting nitric oxide synthase and on their adjacent cells. Nitric oxide can also promote tissues' acute inflammatory response and participate in healing tissue injury and wounds. A moderate amount of nitric oxide can help in the regulation of immune response, while an excessive amount will promote the immune pathological process, which leads to tissue injury. Regulation of nitric oxide levels is helpful for the treatment of many autoimmune diseases.

Nitric oxide helps to resist fatigue

Fatigue is a process that involves a series of complex biochemical changes incurring in the body. The International Sports Biochemical Conference defined fatigue as the point at which an organic physiological process fails to maintain normal function at a given level or when different organs fail to maintain their specified exercise intensity. Fatigue is a protective response that prevents the body from experiencing any excessive functional failure that threatens life. In the event of any fatigue, prompts are issued to reduce working intensity immediately or cease exercise in order to avoid any body injury.

While the body experiences high-intensity exercise, severe ischemia and hypoxia will occur; meanwhile, a greater level of motion will also lead to the re-allocation of blood supply for various tissues in different parts of the body. Blood supply is closely associated with the supply of oxygen as well as nutritional substances and the excretion of metabolites. Therefore, the sports medical circle has also begun to promote the anti-ischemia and hypoxia capacity of the body as one of the most effective methods of promoting exercise capacity and fatigue resistance in the body.

Fatigue is closely related to nitric oxide. In the peripheral fatigue mechanism, high levels of nitric oxide can dilate skeletal muscle vessels, ensure the increase of skeletal muscle blood flow, reduce oxygen consumption, maintain a relatively high oxygen intake rate and yield benefits by delaying the incidence of exercise fatigue. In the central nervous system, nitric oxide can reduce the release of brain endothelin-1 mRNA (ET-lmRNA) due to comparatively intensified exercise load so as to improve cerebral partial ischemia and hypoxia response and provide benefits in regulating the incidence of central fatigue. Due to the double-effect of nitric oxide, replenishment of nitric oxide for the body can play a role in resisting fatigue.

Chapter Seventeen
Nitric oxide and alopecia

Introduction

Hair provides some cranial cushioning and shielding from the sun's rays, and helps to transmit sensory information. Hair is imbued with greater social and psychological significance than with biological importance. It not only plays a vital role in the appearance of both men and women, but also helps to create gender identification and social interaction.

Hair has two distinct structures, the follicle and the shaft, which is what is visible above the scalp. By week 22, a developing fetus has all of its hair follicles formed. This is the largest number of hair follicles a human will ever have, since we do not generate new hair follicles anytime during the course of our lives.

The hair follicle remodels itself during cyclical periods of growth, anagen, catagen, and telogen. Anagen is the active phase of the hair. The cells in the root of the hair are dividing rapidly. The catagen phase is a transitional stage and about 3% of all hairs are in this phase at any time. This phase lasts for about two to three weeks. Telogen is the resting phase and usually accounts for 6% to 8% of all hairs. During this phase, the hair follicle is completely at rest.

Alopecia can be caused by many factors from genetics to the environment. Most common forms of hair loss (alopecia) are caused by aberrant hair follicle cycling and changes in hair follicle morphology.

Androgenetic alopecia (AGA) is by far the most common form of hair loss. And the most common non-AGA alopecias are telogen effluvium, alopecia areata, ringworm, scarring alopecia, and hair loss due to cosmetic overprocessing.

Current treatments

The three distinct aims of therapy for male androgenetic alopecia are: to arrest further progression, to stimulate regrowth and to conceal the hair loss. While successful treatment of hair loss is greatly dependent on early intervention, it is critical to begin treatment with an effective product as soon as you notice the onset of hair loss.

The treatment of hair loss diseases is sometimes difficult because of insufficient efficacy and limited options. Twenty years ago, there were neither specific treatments available for pattern hair loss nor full understanding of the pathophysiology of this common disorder.

It has been widely accepted that topical minoxidil and oral finasteride provide effective remedies for AGA.

Minoxidil was first used in tablet form as a medicine to treat high blood pressure (an antihypertensive). It was noticed that patients being treated with minoxidil experienced excessive hair growth (hypertrichosis) as a side effect. Minoxidil was the first drug approved by the FDA for the treatment of male pattern baldness. For many years, minoxidil, in pill form, was widely used to treat high blood pressure. Women with diffuse androgenetic alopecia can use minoxidil and it actually seems to be more effective for women compared to men. The makers of minoxidil recommend women only use the 2% concentration of minoxidil.

Propecia is the first drug in history to effectively treat male pattern baldness in the vast majority of men who use it. Finasteride's hair-raising success is due to its ability to specifically inhibit Type II 5-alpha-reductace, the enzyme that converts testosterone into a more potent androgen dihydrotestosterone (DHT).

Nitric oxide gel applied topically

These systemic treatments (a pill or other form of internal treatment that affects your entire system) may lower the body's androgen levels. And physicians often choose topical treatments (those that are applied directly to the scalp).

Endogenously produced nitric oxide (NO) has a remarkably diverse range of biological functions, including a role in neurotransmission, smooth muscle relaxation, and the response to immunogens.

Constitutive, low level NO production in the skin seems to play a role in the maintenance of barrier function and in determining blood flow rate in the microvasculature.

Minoxidil, the first drug approved by the FDA for the treatment of male pattern baldness, contains the nitric oxide chemical moiety and its mechanism to promote hair growth is not fully understood. Minoxidil is a potassium channel opener, causing hyperpolarization of cell membranes, and also a vasodilator. Hypothetically, by widening blood vessels and opening potassium channels, it allows more oxygen, blood, and nutrients to the follicle. This may cause follicles in the telogen phase to shed, which are then replaced by thicker hairs in a new anagen phase.

The most common adverse reactions of the topical formulation are limited to irritant and allergic contact dermatitis on the scalp. There have been cases of allergic reactions to the nonactive ingredient propylene glycol, which is found in some topical solution especially if they are galenic. Rarely, cardiovascular side effects have included edema, chest pain, blood pressure changes, palpitations, and changes in pulse rate with minoxidil topical therapy. Despite low levels of systemic absorption, in one study of 35 men using either topical minoxidil 2% twice a day or placebo for 6 months, minoxidil was associated with cardiac changes, such as significant increases in left ventricular end-diastolic volume, cardiac output, and left ventricular mass. Nonspecific allergic reactions, hives, allergic rhinitis, facial swelling, and sensitivity to minoxidil topical have rarely been reported. Headache, dizziness, faintness, and light-headedness, diarrhea, nausea, and vomiting have been reported during treatment with minoxidil topical. Visual disturbances, including decreased visual acuity, have been reported.

Nitric oxide dilates the blood vessels on the area where it is topically applied, which will supposedly stimulate the hair to grow. The dilated blood vessels are also said to absorb more oxygen and nutrients needed for proper hair growth.

As all we know hair follicle density is the key of hair growth. And also the stem cells in bulge that can generate the new hair follicle during cycling and repair the epidermis on injury. In our experiment of effect of NO-gel on wound bed skin of mouse, we found that, compared with the control group, number of hair follicle and stem cell which generate hair follicle in the wound bed in NO treatment group increased significantly.

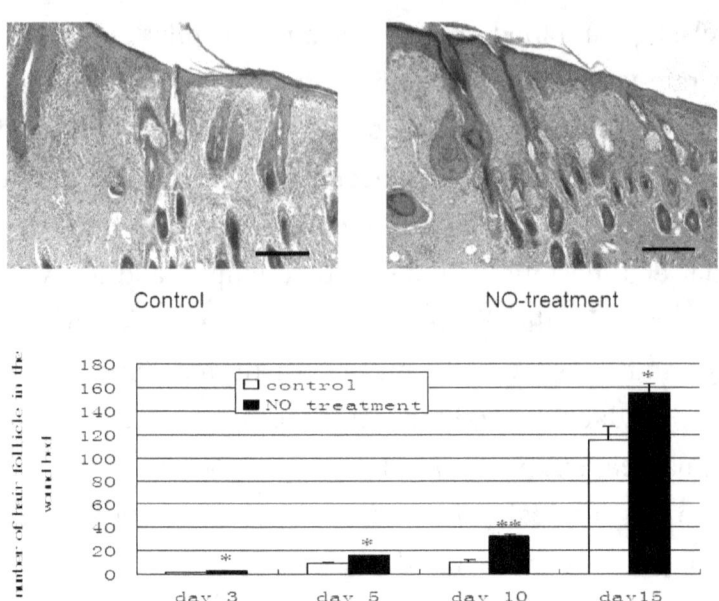

Fig.1 Effect of NO treatment on the number of hair follicle in the wound bed of mouse

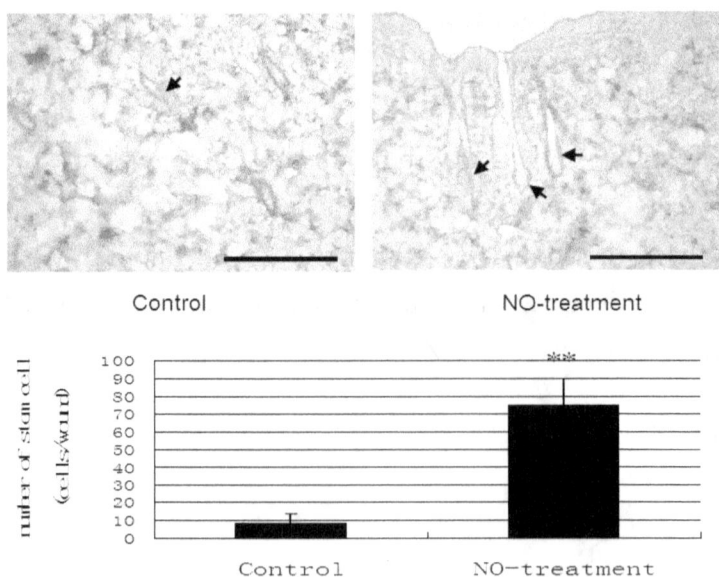

Fig.2 Effect of NO treatment on the number of stem cell in the wound bed of mouse

128

The hair density is dependent on the density of hair follicles. Fig.1 shows that the NO treatment can enhance the number of hair follicle significantly starting from day 5; and on day 15, there was an increase of approximately 35%. The stem cells, containing in the bulge, can generate new hair follicle during cycling and repair of the epidermis after injury. Fig 2 demonstrated the number of stem cells of NO treatment group is 8 times more than that of the control group. These substantial data bring light to the current knowledge and findings on hair follicle research and science.

PART FOUR
"3A & 1S" HEALTHCARE METHODS TO LET YOU LIVE ANOTHER 30 YEARS

In 1998, Dr Murad and other scientists won the Nobel Prize for proving that nitric oxide can have an effect on the human body and is an important signal molecule to regulate blood pressure and blood flow and has an important therapeutic effect for various diseases of the human body. Upon exploration for more than three decades, the international R&D team headed by Dr. Murad has successfully applied nitric oxide technology to food science and technology and proposed the health-keeping method of "three acquisitions and one supplement" (3A & 1S), benefiting even more people in preventing and curing cardio-cerebrovascular diseases and regulating human health. The effects of nitric oxide in the human body have been widely recognized. Nitric oxide can be acquired in such ways as food, moderate exercise and supplements of functional food, while appropriate supplements of antioxidants is another important method to keep nitric oxide formation increased. Therefore, the health-keeping method of "three acquisitions and one supplement" ensures adequate supply of nitric oxide for the body as well as avoids nitric oxide being removed due to rapid oxidation so that the body is always in a healthy state. Therefore, it is accepted by the public and widely applied and highly praised. With time passing, we get older and older. It has always been one of the lasting subjects for man to explore the secret of aging, discover health-keeping methods and seek good medicine for longer healthy life. Everyone wishes for a good health and longevity. Our ancestors have drawn a beautiful blueprint of "living to 120 years, or at least

130

80" for us currently. With more medical research and therapies life expectancy will slowly increase each decade.

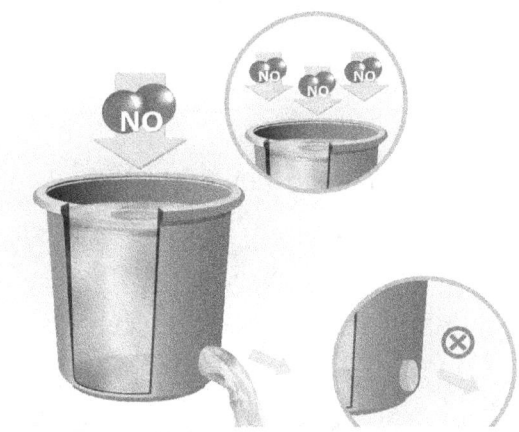

The concentration of cGMP in human body changes dynamically. Stable cGMP concentration and its biochemical reactions not only depend on its generation speed, but also depends on its metabolic rate. The key factor that affects the production of cGMP is guanylate cyclase (GC), and the key factor that affects the metabolic rate of nitric oxide is phosphodiesterase (PDE).

cGMP is catalyzed by guanylate cyclase and produced from GTP, and its hydrolyzation is catalyzed by phosphodiesterase.

Thus there are two ways to increase the concentration of cGMP in human body, that are 1) to activate guanylate cyclase and increase cGMP production or 2) to inhibit phosphodiesterase and slow down the hydrolysis of cGMP. The first mechanism increases the concentration of nitric oxide in the body by orally taking functional food supplement; nitric oxide activates guanylate cyclase. One famous example of the second mechanism is demonstrated by the famous drug "Viagra"; the active ingredient Sildenafil in Viagra inhibits the activity of phosphodiesterase.

Chapter One
Acquisition of Nitric Oxide from Food

Foodstuffs that are rich in nitric oxide

The energy and nutritional substances necessary for maintaining a healthy human body each day are mostly acquired from food. Yet some say "most illnesses are caused by oral consumption", but the smart one can maintain the balance between physical energy and

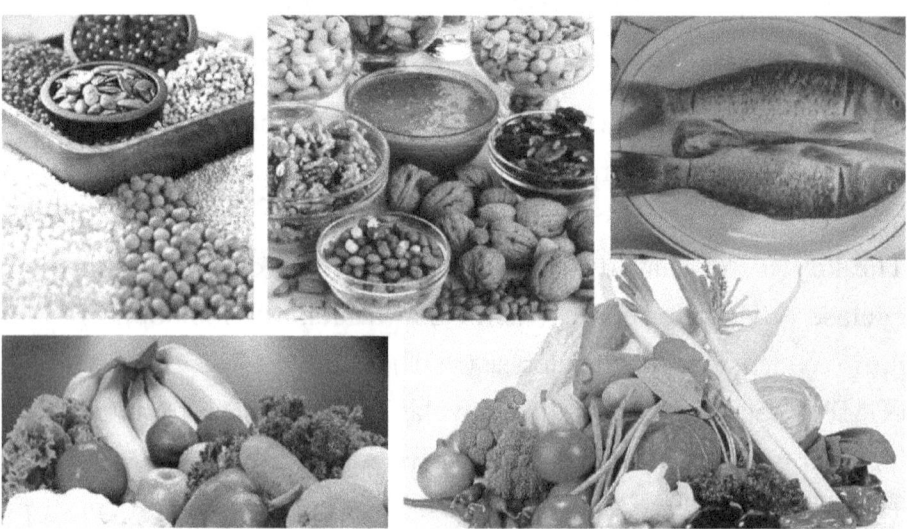

nutritional substances and keep physically healthy through scientific and rational diet, and a balanced calorie intake and expenditure of calories with exercise. Rational diet is also an important approach for us to get nitric oxide.

Major nutritional foodstuffs rich in nitric oxide are:

Cereals and their products yams and their products dry beans and their products, vegetables and their products, fruits and their products, hard nuts and seeds, some animal meats and their products, eggs and their products, fish, prawns, crab and shellfish, dried peeled shrimp (sea shrimp and shelled shrimp) dried razor clam, scallops (dried), cuttlefish (dried), broad-bean sauce and sesame butter.

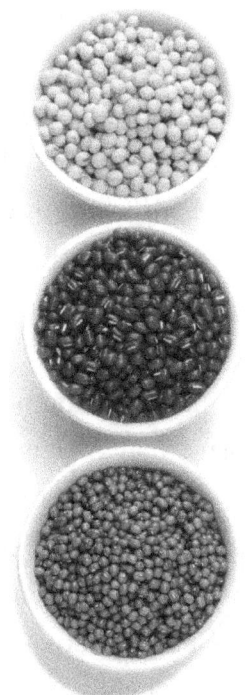

Foodstuffs beneficial for the health of blood and vessels

1) Auricularia: with the effect of preventing aggregation of platelets and resisting coagulation, auricularia can reduce blood aggregation, prevent the formation of thrombus, and delay the incidence and development of atherosclerosis. Garlic polysaccharide in auricularia can also regulate blood lipids.

Auricularia with added crystal sugar can lower blood pressure and

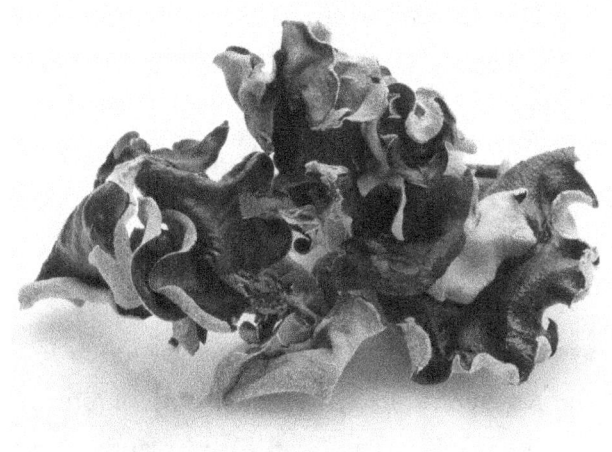

prevent vascular sclerosis. Consumed frequently together with garlic and scallions, auricularia can relieve coronary artery atherosclerosis. Take 15g of auricularia daily for cooking soup or frying.

2) Shiitake: including oyster mushroom, straw mushroom, etc., all of which are high-protein and low-fat healthy foods rich in vitamins. In particular, shiitake also has the effect of lowering blood pressure, as it contains nucleic acid substances that inhibit the production of cholesterol, they prevent lipids from attaching themselves to the arterial wall, and prevent atherosclerosis and brittle vessels in order to ensure that vessels remain young and pliable.

3) Honey: contains Vitamin C, Vitamin K, Vitamin B_2, Vitamin B_6, carotene; and is able to improve blood circulation of coronary vessels, and prevents vascular sclerosis.

4) Chinese dates: contain abundant Vitamin P, Vitamin P enhances capillary elasticity and prevents hemorrhagic diseases.

5) Eggplant: contains Vitamin P, especially purple eggplant, which has the highest content. Vitamin P can enhance the elasticity of capillaries. Eggplant also contains Vitamin A, Vitamin C, protein and calcium, which can soften human vessels. It can also reduce the probability of cardiovascular thrombus formation. Therefore, eggplant is important to the prevention and treatment of hypertension, artery atherosclerosis and cerebral strokes.

6) Tomato: contains Vitamin P, which can protect vessels and control hypertension. Lycopene and cellulose in tomatoes have the effect of lowering cholesterol and metabolizing alkaloids, so as to stop human atherosclerosis and prevent the incidence of coronary heart disease.

7) Sweet potato: contains a mixture of polysaccharide and protein; consuming in larger quantities can reduce the content of cholesterol in the blood, and it is highly beneficial for preventing and controlling

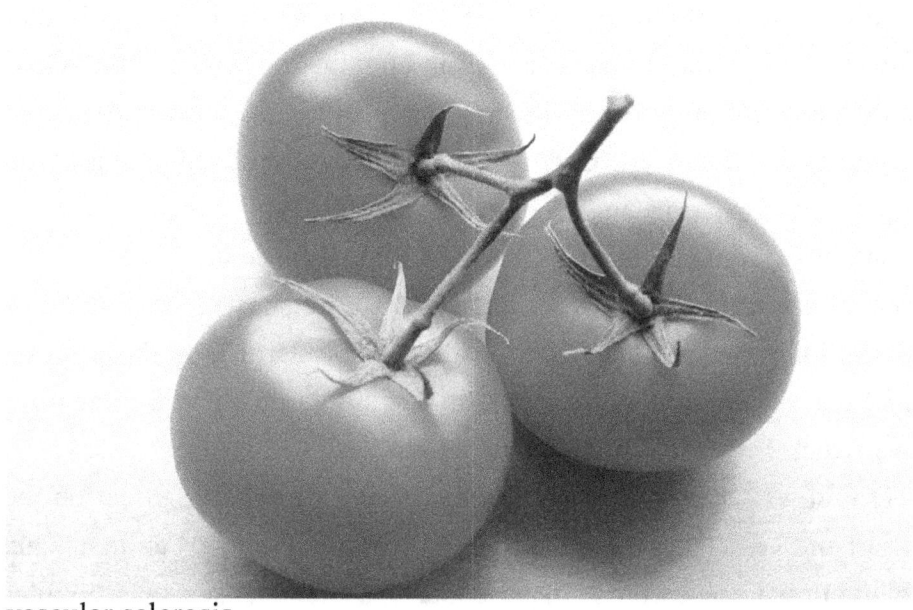

vascular sclerosis.

8) Corn: rich in protein, with unsaturated fatty acids (mainly linoleic acid and oleic acid) of up to 85% or more; contains large quantities of lecithin, calcium, phosphorus, selenium and other trace elements as well as Vitamin E, etc., with the effects of preventing cellular rupture, delaying cellular aging, lowering serum cholesterol, preventing skin lesions, as well as demonstrating a positive effect in relieving atherosclerosis and cerebral function failure.

9) Onion: contains prostaglandins, which dilate vessels and regulate blood lipids, preventing artery atherosclerosis and avoiding the formation or prevention of thrombus. Onion contains essential oils, which can regulate blood lipids. Onion is the only known plant that contains prostaglandin A, which is a relatively strong type of vasodilator that can relax vessels, lower blood viscosity, and increase blood flow in the coronary arteries, with the effect of reducing and preventing the formation of thrombus.

10) Garlic: contains a mixture of sulfides, which not only reduce cholesterol in blood, but also can quickly drive away lipids that attach to the arterial vascular wall in conjunction with the flavonoid substance contained therein, thereby preventing the incidence of coronary heart disease. Garlic also has the effect of regulating blood lipids and resisting aggregation of platelets, and can increase the content of HDL useful for health, which significantly reduces the risk of coronary heart disease. As studies have shown, fresh garlic or garlic juice can prevent rising levels of cholesterol to high-fat meals and can eliminate the accumulation of lipids on the vascular inter wall, thereby decreasing atherosclerosis.

11) Ginger: contains gingerol, which has a stimulating effect on the heart and vessels, causing the heart to beat faster, vessels to dilate, and blood flow to accelerate. Ginger contains a chemical substance similar to salicylic acid, which can prevent blood coagulation, and is highly efficient at regulating blood lipid and blood pressure and preventing thrombus. Additionally, ginger also contains a kind of oleoresin, which has the significant effect on the regulation of blood lipid and reduction of cholesterol.

12) Kelp and seaweed: rich in taurine, which reduces cholesterol in the blood and bile; the alginic acid thereof also can inhibit the absorption of cholesterol and promote metabolism. Kelp is a polysaccharide and can reduce the content of serum cholesterol and triglyceride. What is more, these foodstuffs are also rich in various essential amino acids.

13) Walnut: containing linoleic acid, another unsaturated fatty acid; linoleic acid causes the body to excrete cholesterol and make it uneasy for surplus cholesterol to be absorbed, thereby limiting atherosclerosis. Walnut is also rich in phosphorus, and provides nutrition to the cranial nerves; if three walnuts are consumed daily, the level of cholesterol in the blood can be reduced by 5% and the risk for cardiovascular diseases can be reduced by 10%.

14) Chinese hawthorn: many nutrients present in Chinese hawthorn can have the effect of strengthening the heart, dilating vessels, increasing coronary arterial blood flow and reducing pressure as well as regulating blood lipids by improving blood circulation and promoting the excretion of cholesterol. Chinese hawthorn can significantly reduce the content of serum cholesterol and triglyceride thereby effectively controlling atherosclerosis. Chinese hawthorn also can increase myocardial contractility and dilate coronary arterial vessels. However, individuals suffering from an excess of gastric acid are advised not to ingest Chinese hawthorn. Gastric and duodenal ulcer patients with ulcers for a long time also should not take Hawthorn.

15) Apple: apples are rich in polysaccharides, flavonoids, potassium, Vitamin C and other nutritional components, which can decompose fatty acid in the body, avoid obesity and reduce burdens on the heart. Flavonoid substances contained in apples are natural antioxidants, which can decrease atherosclerosis by inhibiting LDL oxidation.

16) Beans: soybean is not only a good source of protein, but also a healthy food for preventing lipid abnormality and coronary heart disease. With extremely low sugar, it is suitable for consumption by diabetic patients. Soybeans contain rich unsaturated fatty acid, Vitamin E, and lecithin, which regulate blood lipid levels. Therefore, it is beneficial for patients with hypercholesterolemia to eat soybeans and related products.

17) Oats: oleic acid, linoleic acid, saponin, lecithin and calcium, magnesium, selenium and other inorganic salts are all present in oats and are capable of reducing deposits of serum cholesterol on arterial walls so as to prevent atherosclerosis. It contains linoleic acid, which accounts for 35%~52% of the total unsaturated fatty acid. It has a high content of Vitamin E and saponin, which can reduce total cholesterol levels and triglyceride, as well as clear LDL on the vascular wall and prevent atherosclerosis.

18) Fish: fish contains various unsaturated fatty acids necessary for the human body, which inhibit platelet aggregation and reduce cholesterol. Sea fish oil also contains relatively large quantities of unsaturated fat. As clinical studies indicate, individuals that consume more fish will experience a reduction in plasma lipids. Therefore, frequent consumption of fish can prevent atherosclerosis.

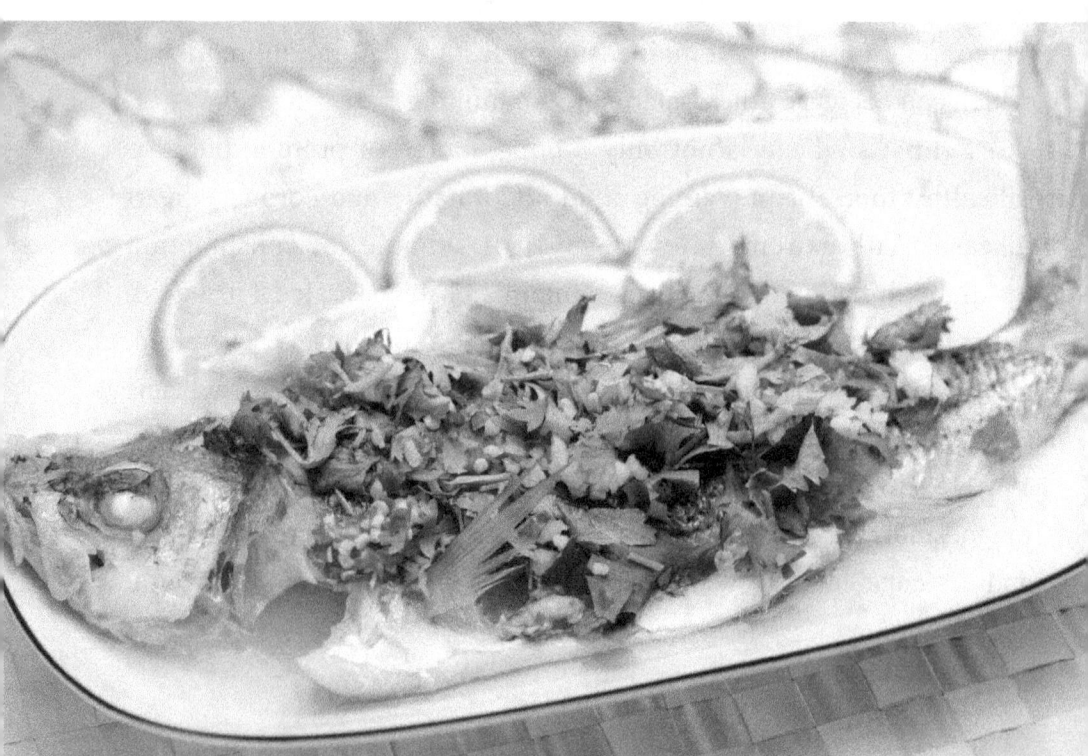

19) Chrysanthemum: chrysanthemum helps to regulate blood lipid as well as exerting a very stable effect to lower blood pressure. A small amount of chrysanthemum added to green tea will yield potent benefits to the well-being of the heart and vessels, especially for the middle-aged and elderly.

20) Tea: contains tea polyphenol, which can improve the antioxidation capacity of the body as well as regulate blood lipids, relieve high blood concentration, enhance the elasticity of erythrocytes, and relax or delay arterial atherosclerosis. Frequent drinking of tea may also soften arterial vessels.

21) Kumquat: kumquat is rich in Vitamin C, which can accelerate the transformation of cholesterol and play a role in regulating blood lipids and relieving atherosclerosis. Kumquat also contains kumquat glycoside and other substances, which can reduce the brittleness and permeability of capillaries, relieve vascular sclerosis, and regulate blood pressure.

22) Red Sweet potato: sweet potato is rich in potassium, carotene, folic acid, Vitamin C and Vitamin B_6, all of which are helpful for the prevention of atherosclerosis. Carotene and Vitamin C have the effect of resisting the oxidation of lipids and preventing arterial atherosclerosis. Supplemented with folic acid and Vitamin B_6, it is helpful to lower the level of cysteine in blood and prevent the injury of arterial vessels. It also provides significant quantities of collagen and mucopolysaccharide substances that help maintain the elasticity of arterial vessels.

23) Cherry: able to clear toxins from the human body, especially in the kidney, as well as producing the effect of catharsis.

24) Grape: in particular, dark purple grapes have the effect of removing toxins, which help to clear the refuse in the liver, intestine, stomach and kidney.

25) Strawberry: strawberry can remove toxins, and can help clean the gastrointestinal tract.

Fruits can increase the production of NO, increase antioxidation and decrease the consumption of NO

Fruits which can increase production of nitric oxide in vivo
Hawthorn: with obvious hypolipemic effects and the effect of increasing NO production, hawthorn plays an important role in protecting vascular endothelial cells and preventing and curing cardiovascular and cerebrovascular diseases. With antioxidatiive properties, the Vitamin C contained in hawthorn can effectively scavenge in vivo oxygen radicals, preventing NO levels from declining and maintaining the biological activity of NO.

Grape: Grape phytochemicals such as anthocyanin, resveratrol, vitamin C and vitamin E, all are antioxidants, and can remove ROS that inhibit nitric oxide production.

Researchers have discovered that although the French tend to eat higher levels of animal fat, the incidence of heart disease remains low in France. It is thought to occur from the protective benefits of regularly consuming red wine, with a polyphenol antioxidant— resveratrol in grapes.

Synthesized by many plants, resveratrol apparently has antifungal and other defensive properties. Dietary resveratrol has been shown to modulate the metabolism of lipids to inhibit oxidation of low-density lipoproteins and the aggregation of platelets.

Resveratrol enhances endothelial NO production by reducing the cofactors for NOS and increasing eNOS enzyme activity and it also lowers endothelial levels of ROS which degrade NO.

Date: date contains rutin which helps slow down brain aging. Possibly by increasing the activity of NOS, the effect increases the production of endogenous NO, strengthens the removal of free radicals which increase with age, and retards lipid peroxidation. The Vitamin A and Vitamin C found in dates are important antioxidants.

Fruits which can increase antioxidation and decrease the consumption of NO

Kiwi fruit: one kiwi fruit can provide more than two times the amount of Vitamin C required for one person per day. It is for this reason that kiwi fruit is honored as the "King of Fruits". Vitamin C is an extremely strong antioxidant and can scavenge in vivo oxygen radicals, prevent NO levels from declining and maintaining the biological activity of NO.

Sour jujube: sour jujube contains Vitamin C, Vitamin E, sour jujube amylase and sour jujube polyphenols. Sour jujube extracts are an extremely strong antioxidant and can scavenge in vivo oxygen radicals, preventing NO levels from declining and maintaining the biological activity of NO.

Apple: malic acid, and sufficient amounts of polyphenols and Vitamin C found in apples can enhance antioxidant capacity and can scavenge in vivo oxygen radicals, preventing NO levels from declining and maintaining the biological activity of NO.

Orange: orange is rich in antioxidants such as hesperidin, aurantiin and Vitamin C, which resist oxidation and eliminate free radicals and can prevent NO levels from declining and help maintain the biological activity of NO.

Lemon: lemon is one of the fruits with the most medicinal value in the world and is rich in Vitamin C, citric acid, malic acid, hesperidin, aurantin and so on, which are extremely strong antioxidants and can eliminate in vivo oxygen radicals, preventing NO levels from declining and maintaining the biological activity of NO.

Blueberry: blueberry contains Vitamin A, Vitamin C and Vitamin E, which are extremely strong antioxidants, and can eliminate in vivo oxygen radicals, preventing NO levels from declining and maintaining the biological activity of NO.

Cherry and pomelo: cherry and pomelo both contain Vitamin C, which can eliminate in vivo oxygen radicals, prevent NO levels from declining, and maintain the biological activity of NO.

Man and arteries have the same lifetime

As the famous 19th century French doctor Kasabian, once said, "Man and arteries have the same lifetime". This means that human arteries continue to be hardened and blocked until the important organs (heart and brain) become infarcted and necrotic and human life eventually ends. As the human body ages, vessels will naturally degenerate. Vascular aging causes the blood supply and oxygen supply of the systemic tissues to become blocked, which is represented physically by walking difficulties, by numbness in the limbs and slow reaction by tissue and organs as well as by coronary heart disease and cerebral stroke. Therefore to preserve the health of the human body, it is critical to delay the process of vascular sclerosis. As long as we attach importance to a scientific diet, improving dietary structure, enhancing physical exercise and sustaining healthy living habits vascular sclerosis can be slowed and even reversed.

Chapter Two
Acquisition of Nitric Oxide from Healthy Exercise

Persist in regular physical activities

Nitric oxide is closely associated with physical motion. It can dilate skeletal muscle vessels, ensure the increase of metabolic skeletal muscle blood flow, reduce the oxygen consumption of skeletal muscle and promote the transport of glucose into skeletal muscle cells.

Short-term acute exercise can cause a sharp increase in nitric oxide generation. Short-term acute exercise promotes the release of nitric oxide possibly because when exercising blood flow speeds up, after sport this can relax blood vessels by an endothelium-dependent manner and the increase of shear stress can active the NOS-3 in endothelium cells. With the density of calcium ions in skeletal muscle cells increasing, it continues to activate the calcium-dependent nitric oxide synthase. Lasting physical exercise can up-regulate the expression of messenger RNA and increase the capacity of endothelium and skeletal muscle to generate nitric oxide.

As the human body reaches middle age, vessels will continue to age, which will lead to cardio-cerebrovascular diseases. By persisting in regular physical activities, the body will continue to produce nitric oxide, so as to gradually delay the progress of vascular aging. Nowadays, the hazards of atherosclerosis are known to everyone; atherosclerosis is the basic cause for coronary heart disease, hypertension, and cerebral strokes and is a direct or indirect high-risk factor for many diseases that afflict the elderly such as cardiovascular diseases, diabetes and dementia. For a long time, researchers have

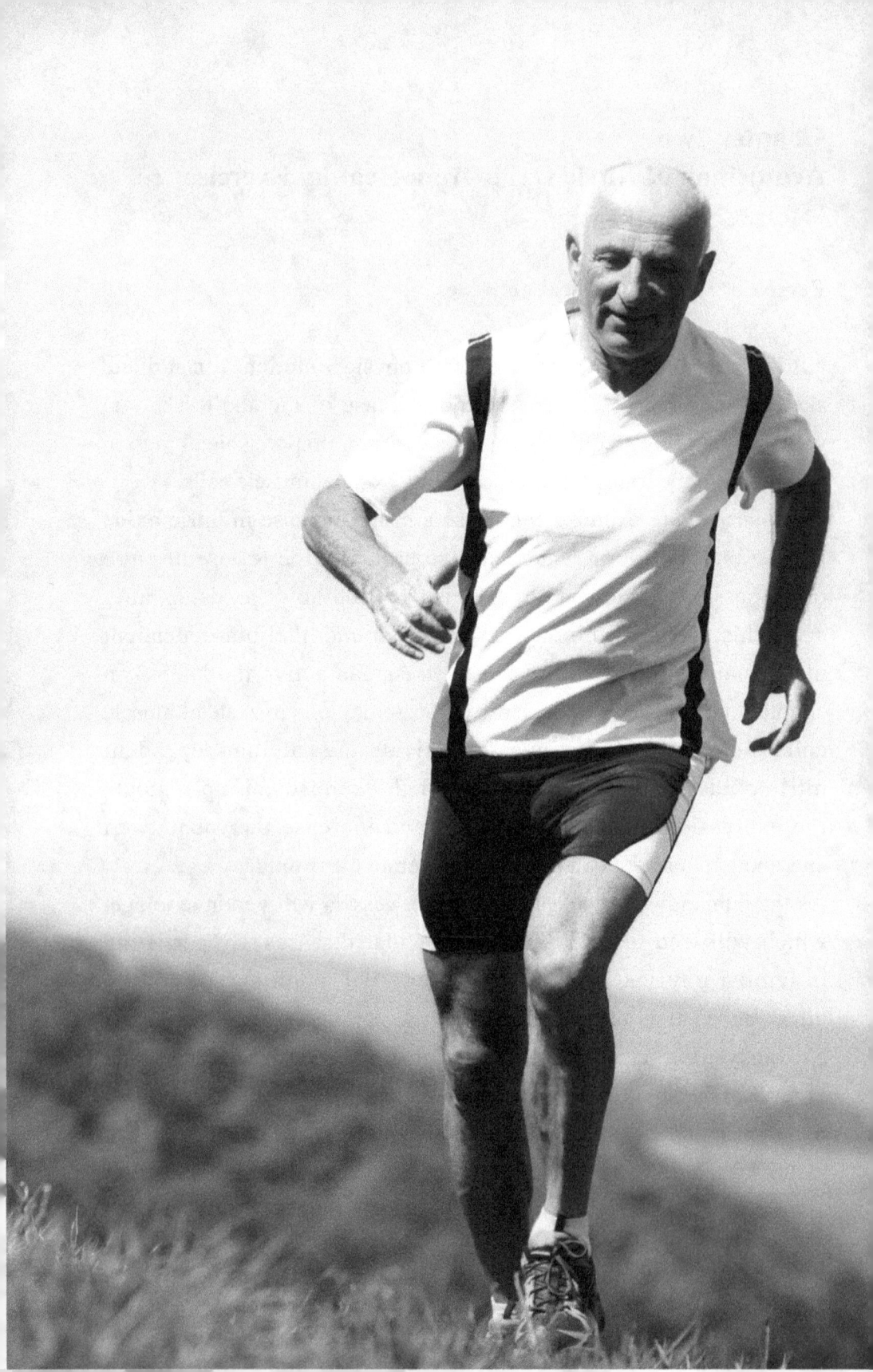

had no idea about how to cope with such a killer. Atherosclerosis has always been considered an inevitable effect of the natural aging process. As the studies of applied medicine in recent years have discovered, people have found the method for governing and even reversing it: exercise.

Life relies on exercise and so do vessels. The American Heart Association conducted comparative research on young (with an average age of 27 years) and old athletes (with an average age of 65 years), of which the results indicated that long-term regular physical activities or exercises can protect human vascular endothelium, avoid vascular aging due to the growing age, and keep the vascular function of the elders as good as that of young people. According to the further research, the level of free radicals in the blood of old athletes was as low as that of the younger participants, while elderly people not fond of exercising showed a relatively high level of free radicals.

Why can exercise keep vessels young? One of the secrets is that exercise can promote the level of in vivo HDL, commonly known as good cholesterol. "Good cholesterol" is good for its small, high density granules, which can freely access and exit arterial vascular walls to clear LDL deposited on vessels thereby avoiding erosion on arterial walls. For this reason, HDL is known as a "cleaner" of vessels.

As research data shows, exercising for half an hour daily, such as walking, riding a bike, swimming, playing gate ball, playing table tennis, jogging, climbing stairs or mountains, can be effective in reducing weight and burning fat to increase the young life span of vessels and prevent vascular aging.

Foods containing comparatively large quantities of fat can increase the level of blood lipids for the time being as well as cause injuries to the function of vascular endothelium, while exercise can minimize such injuries. According to the latest research, strolling for a relatively long distance before ingesting large quantities of oily food can reduce the harm of fat to vascular functions.

Effect of exercise on different major systems

In the 18th century, the French doctor, Tisso said: "so far as its effect is concerned, exercise can act as a substitute for almost all drugs, but no drugs in the world can substitute for the effect of exercising." This expression has vividly outlined the effect of exercising on health. Moderate exercise is a good medicine for heath as well as a major approach for endothelial cells to produce nitric oxide. Participation in healthy exercise activities can have direct, beneficial effects on multiples systems within the body:

1) Cardiovascular system: exercise can enhance the functions of the cardiovascular system. For lovers of exercise, myocardial contraction strengthens, blood circulation increases, the diameter of the coronary artery that supplies nutrition to the heart becomes larger, blood supply to the heart improves, the elasticity of systemic vessels is enhanced, artery atherosclerosis is delayed, cardiac function is enhanced, adaptation of blood pressure and heart rate to different conditions is also enhanced.

2) Respiratory system: exercise can improve respiratory function. Since the human body needs to absorb a considerable amount of oxygen and release a correspondingly large amount of CO_2 when exercising, vital capacity increases and residual volume decreases, thus allowing pulmonary function to be enhanced. A well-functioning respiratory system is highly beneficial to the human body, allowing it to remain vigorous and postponing the aging process.

3) Digestive system: exercise can improve the function of the digestive system. Because humans need to consume certain energy when exercising, exercise enhances the rate of consumption of in vivo nutritional substances as well as the metabolism of the whole body, thus increasing the appetite. Exercise also promotes gastrointestinal peristalsis and secretion of digestive fluid, improving the functions of the liver and pancreas, thus improving the efficiency of the whole digestive system and assuring the continuous supply of health-giving substances to the body.

4) Nervous system: exercise may improve nervous system function. Since exercising is a coordinative activity controlled by the nervous system, elderly individuals that persevere with exercise activities often demonstrate a flexible body, good hearing and vision facilities, and high energy levels. Exercise can promote cerebral blood circulation, improve the oxygen and nutrition supply to cerebral cells, delay the aging process of the central nervous system, and increase its working efficiency. This is extremely important for people working in cognitively intensive fields. The repetition of muscle activity and exercise further improves the regulatory capacity of the nervous system, which in turn regulates the function of cerebral cortex. In particular, light exercise may mitigate tension in the nerves and help to prevent conditions such as neurosis, emotional depression, insomnia, hypertension, and so on.

5) Motion system: exercise develops muscles. Exercise may improve the contraction and relaxation capacity of muscles and make muscle fiber thicker and muscle strength greater. Exercise can improve systemic blood circulation as well as nutrition levels in muscles and the skeleton, enhance the metabolism of the skeleton, and increase the skeleton's elasticity and toughness, thus delaying the aging process and preventing such symptoms as osteoporosis, bone joint degeneration and joint pain.

6) Endocrine system: exercise has a great effect on the endocrine system, especially the pituitary gland, and is important for the regulation of metabolism functions in the adrenal system, pancreas and other digestive glands. Positive changes in physical structure and function due to long-term exercising, provides a healthy and strong skeleton, toughness of the ligaments, elasticity of vessels, thickening of myocardium, and increase of capillary networks, are all possible thanks to the regulation of the endocrine system. Exercise can improve glucose metabolism and control diabetes, can bring down serum cholesterol, prevent atherosclerosis, promote the metabolism of surplus fat and prevent obesity. It can also improve sexual function and enhance sexual life. All these are related to improvements in the regulating function of the endocrine system.

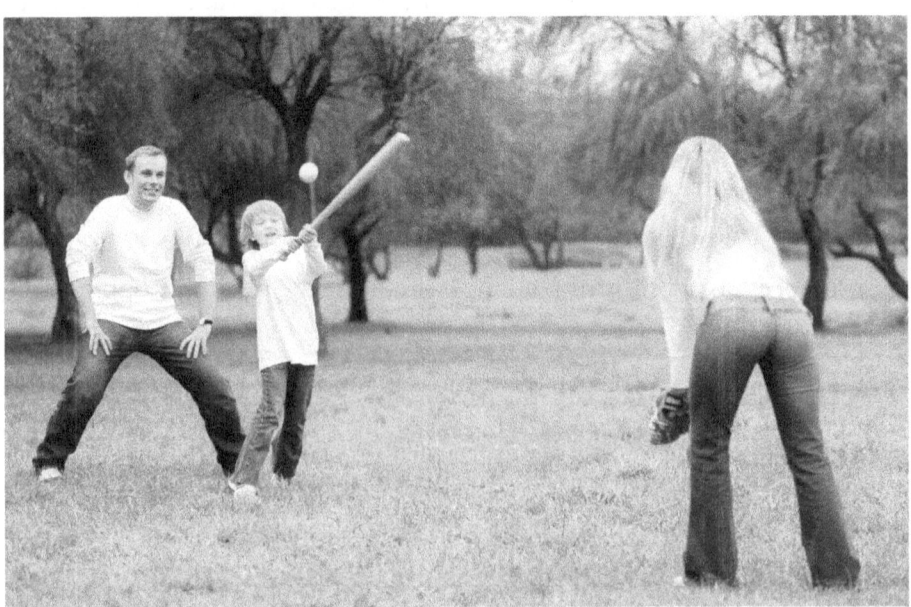

7) Immune system: at present, both Chinese and foreign scholars are in agreement that physical exercise can mobilize the capacity of the human immune system to deal with stress. Through extensive experiments, it has been shown that the aging of the body does not necessarily lead to a decline in the efficiency of immune function.

Scientific and effective exercising methods

Importance of exercising cannot be overstated, but how can we exercise in a scientific way and sustain exercise over a long period of time? Experts have offered the following recommendations:

1) Select a suitable form of exercise

Interest is the best teacher. Many people know about the benefit of exercising, but few people can persist in exercising. According to recommendations by experts, it is best to choose a form of exercise that interests you, as this will help you to sustain a regular activity over a long period of time. All you need to do is persevere in one or two forms of exercise, be they jogging, cycling, swimming, tennis, yoga, dancing, or skipping, and you will soon begin to feel the benefits.

2) Design an exercise plan

This is a good way to monitor your progress and set achievable goals. Set a minimum goal to complete every week, such as 20 minutes of exercise per day, then, gradually increase the intensity of the exercise each week to maximize the physical potential of your body.

3) Regular physical checkups

Tangible results are an excellent incentive for sustaining exercise. Seeing an improvement in key indicators in the physical check-up reports for yourself, will give you a clear idea of your progress and heighten your sense of achievement.

The Physiotherapy of Nitric Oxide - Exercise

As early as 400 BC, the Greek physician Hippocrates, who was widely regarded as the founder of medicine, he once said, "Eating alone will not maintain a man's wellness; he must also exercise. Even though food and exercise possesses opposite functions, the two work together to promote health…".

Actively participate in sport activities is the fundamental basis for maintaining a healthy body.

A large number of studies showed that actively participate in sport activities can effectively reduce the risk of many diseases, such as lowering blood lipid level, regulating blood pressure, regulating blood glucose level and improving bone mineral density.

Many chronic diseases can also be controlled or treated effectively through exercise.

One: The relationship between exercise and nitric oxide

Exercise enhances the capacity of platelets to transit L-arginine; which strengthens the synthesis of nitric oxide (NO). NO can inhibit platelet aggregation, which significantly benefits the health of human body.

Studies showed that long-term exercising can increase NO synthesis and production in vascular endothelial and skeletal muscle.

A research on patients with heart disease showed that, after 6 months of regular exercising, it promotes endothelial NO synthesis, and also encourages the expansion of skeletal muscle depended vascular endothelial.

Clinical practice has proved that chronic heart disease caused by high cholesterol level is related to endothelial function loss and NO synthesis reduction.

Patients with blood vessel embolism disease that are dedicated to exercising can increase the synthesis of NO, which functions on disease prevention and control.

Two: The benefits of exercises on health

As commonly known, exercising is one of the easiest methods to promote and maintain a healthy lifestyle. Dedication to sport activities can make a person feel better both physically and mentally. It helps to keep the flexibility of muscles, strengthens the function of muscles, joints and bones and improves the pumping efficiency of the heart. It also helps to improve blood circulation, prevent cardiovascular disease, and at the same time, relieve stress and depression and improve insomnia and menopausal symptoms.

Exercise and cardiovascular disease

Most research showed a reverse relation between moderate intensity exercise and coronary heart disease. To one's surprise, doctors state that the harm of physical exercise deficiency is more harmful to one's health then mid level coronary heart disease. Studies have shown that the human body promotes the formation of nitric oxide through exercising. Nitric oxide can lower blood pressure and blood lipid level, and improve glucose metabolism. Maintaining an active exercising life style can reduce the systolic blood pressure and diastolic blood pressure, the average cholesterol, triglyceride and low density lipoprotein (LDL) levels. This consequentially raises the high density lipoprotein (HDL) level, and promotes the activity of the cholesterol based transfer enzymes. This in turn increases the HDL2 level, and reduces the risk of developing cardiovascular diseases.

Exercise and diabetes

At the current stage, the pathogenesis of diabetes is not completely understood, however, a large number of research studies proved that long-term exercising lifestyle is beneficial to patients with diabetes.

The mechanical function can be explained as follows: the energy cost for physical activity increases, which strengthens the skeletal muscle to absorb glucose and increases the level of glucose transporters and the glucose transporter proteins in plasma and skeletal muscles. This in turns increases the level of glycogen synthase and increases the release of non-oxidated glucose.

Studies have reported that as people gets older, the risk for less active people to suffer from diabetes increases by 20% or more as compared to regular exercisers.

It showed a stronger protective effect of exercising in susceptibility of obese people to type 2 diabetes as well. Exercises can improves condition of type 1 diabetes patients, and better prevents the development of type 2 diabetes.

Exercise and osteoporosis

Osteoporosis is another kind of chronic diseases that threatens human health.

The etiology of primary osteoporosis is not very clear. Aging and insufficient physical activity is considered to be the most significant cause of bone mineral loss and osteoporosis. Increasing physical activity allows bone formation to increase.

The mechanism of exercises in increasing bone mineral density includes: supplying mechanical force to stimulate bone formation, to activate bone cells and strengthens bone formation.

Long-term exercise habit can reduce blood insulin level, and boost glucagon, catecholamine and thyrotropin levels, thus increasing bone mineral content.

Three: Exercise and health

Dedicating to exercising lifestyle

Benefits to aerobics exercise are countless, it helps to reduce the volume of subcutaneous fat, aid in digestion and increase circulation of blood. Aerobics exercises are usually less strenuous; it is often rhythmic and continuous in nature. Examples for aerobics exercise include: walking, cycling, jogging, swimming, tai chi, etc.

Recommendations for optimal aerobic exercise:
1) to exercise in an oxygen rich environment with good ventilation, exercising outdoors is the best;
2) to exercise for 30~60 consecutive minutes for maximum health effects;
3) to reach a heart rate of less than 150 times/min when exercising.

Preparation for exercise

Every time before commencing exercise, it is essential to perform warm up preparations. Such preparation should include: moderate movement of the upper and lower limb, waist, ankle joints, loosening the muscles on legs and arms; taking a couple deep breaths to allow gas exchange of lungs, and to increase cardio capacity. These prepare the body for a full workout and avoid muscle and ligament injuries.

Control the amount of exercise

People should avoid excessive and strenuous exercises during their workout. Excessive and strenuous exercises are not necessarily better, in some ways, it could even be an disadvantage to one's health. Generally speaking, it is the best to control the amount of exercise in moderate load and intensity. In the beginning of any exercise practice, a large quantity of exercise is unfavorable.

The amount of exercise should be done step by step with gradual increase. After exercise, it is advised that the measured pulse for young people should not exceed 150 per minute, and for the elderly, not to exceed 110 per minute.

The best time to exercise

The best time to exercise is around 7 to 8 pm. It is inappropriate to exercise when one's starved, before meals and before bedtime. When one's determined to maintain an exercise routine, it is important to be consistent.   It has always been a universal goal of mankind to find the secret of longevity and trap youthfulness as long as possible.

Scientific researchers have proved that most people can achieve such goals through consistent exercising. It will not be hard for one to keep a long and healthy life if he or she is determined to consistently incorporate exercising into their lives.

Chapter Three
Acquisition of Nitric Oxide from Functional Food

What is functional food?

"Functional food" is a special kind of food, which is important to ensure the normal functioning of one or more regulatory processes in the body that are necessary to maintain human health. It is therefore normally intended for people with a deficiency in a particular nutrient. Functional food has a more powerful effect on several aspects of human health than ordinary food, but, since it cannot directly treat diseases and has a weaker effect than medicine; the process by which this food regulates human health occurs over a long period of time. In recent years, the functional food industry has developed rapidly throughout the world. Health-care (functional) food is known as "healthy food" or "nutritional food" in Europe and America and as "functional food" in Japan.

At present, China defines health-care products as: food that regulates human physiological function, is suitable for specific groups within the general population, but for the purpose of treatment. In addition to the nutrition and sensory functions (color, fragrance, taste and form) available in normal food, such food also has a third function that is not as prominent in general food: i.e., the regulation of human physiological functions. For this reason, it is known as "functional food".

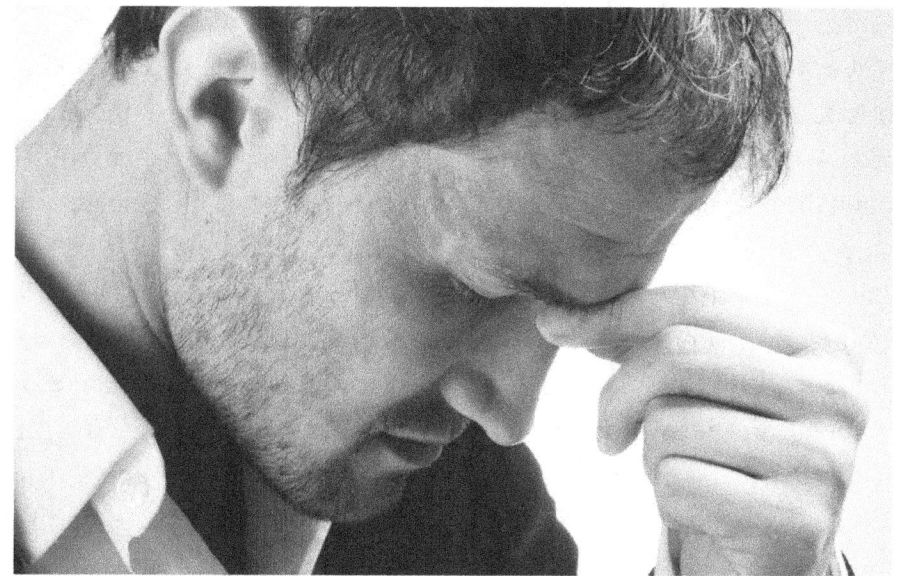
Subhealthy state

It is the opinion of experts in this field that the functional orientation of health-care products should be targeted towards individuals in a state of sub-health (or sub-clinical state). Its purpose should be to regulate, relieve and improve pre-disease conditions in the target groups and pre-emptively ensures that a state of normal health is achieved. Appropriate supplements of functional food rich in nitric oxide have an extremely positive and important role in the prevention and improvement of cardio-cerebrovascular diseases.

NO nutritional supplements

NO nutritional supplements are a kind of functional food that can promote the generation of nitric oxide in the body for a short time period, thereby maintaining the health of blood and vessels. Currently, the main components of NO nutritional supply include: arginine, citrulline and compound vitamins.

L-arginine and L-citrulline are both amino acids, both can be synthesized in the human body through the ingestion of certain kinds of food and through exercise. As the blood and vessels age, the human body will start to supplement such amino acid in large quantities to maintain physical health. At present, the two types of amino acid are called semi-essential amino acids.

Since amino acid is the basic unit of protein, many people consider food rich in protein as lean meat, chicken and fish to be the best source of L-arginine and L-citrulline. However, it is also dangerous to focus on these foods as sources of L-arginine and L-citrulline in daily life, as many foodstuffs rich in such amino acids often contain excessive saturated fatty acid, which will generate harmful cholesterol, and speed up congestion and sclerosis of the vessels. Therefore, a safe method for increasing the intake of such amino acids as L-arginine and L-citrulline is to supplement functional food rich in L-arginine and L-citrulline in moderate amounts. In this way, we can absorb more L-arginine and L-citrulline as well as avoid the intake of high-fat.

When L-arginine is digested in moderate quantities, it will spread throughout the body via the blood circulation. When it enters into the vascular endothelial cells of blood vessel walls, an enzyme reaction changes L-arginine into nitric oxide.

Pomegranate and nitric oxide

Many people enjoy drinking pomegranate juice for its pleasant taste and rich content of vitamin C, which contains twice as much as apple and pear juice. Moreover, pomegranate can reduce the risk of heart disease and help prevent prostate cancer. In ancient Greece, pomegranate was a symbol of fertility. A report showed that pomegranate juice can cure erectile dysfunction and its effect can

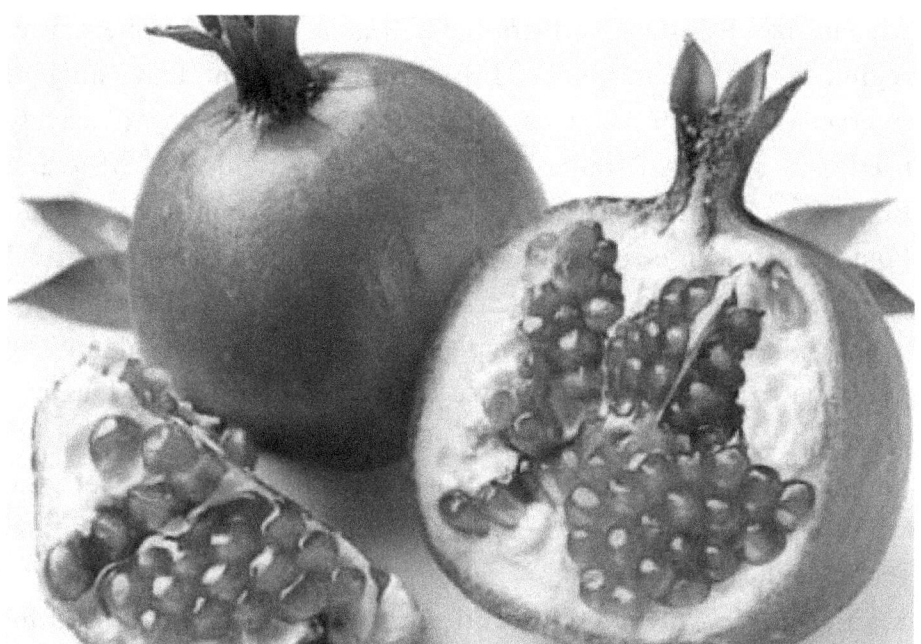

rival that of the famous drug Viagra. According to new research, a daily glass of pomegranate juice could help to protect against male impotence. Men who drank the juice every day for a month reported better performance in the bedroom. The study suggests pomegranate juice could be a drug-free alternative to Viagra.

The level of nitric oxide in the human body is not fixed but in a constant state of fluctuation. Sufficient concentrations of NO necessary for it to fulfill its biological function depend on not only the synthesis rate but also on the catabolic metabolism rate. Factors influencing the synthesis rate include substrates and enzymes of the NO synthesis process. And the redox state of the human body is a major factor effecting catabolic metabolism rate. In addition to containing the NO synthesis substrate, which can induce the expression of eNOS, pomegranate juice is also rich in antioxidants which significantly reduce the oxidation of NO.

The pomegranate is native to the region of Persia and the western Himalayan range, and has been cultivated in Iran, Azerbaijan,

Afghanistan, Pakistan, Northern India, Russia, and the Mediterranean region for several millennia. In the Indian subcontinent's ancient Ayurveda system of medicine, the pomegranate has been extensively used as a source of traditional remedies for thousands of years. Pomegranate contains plenty of polyphenols and flavones. Pomegranate can effectively scavenge superoxide anion, hydroxyl radical, and lipid peroxy radical, and can inhibit oxidation of low density lipoprotein. Pomegranate is an effective antioxidant. The polyphenols found in pomegranate juice are antioxidants, which can lower oxidative stress and delay atherosclerosis.

Pomegranate juice can prevent the oxidation of NO, protect the vascular endothelium, activate eNOS and enhance the biological action of NO.

Studies indicate that both extracts of pomegranate fruit and pomegranate juice can activate the expression of eNOS, enhance the synthesis of NO and promote NO levels. Pomegranate juice concentrate reduces the activation of redox-sensitive genes (ELK-1 and p-JUN) and increased eNOS expression (which was decreased by perturbed shear stress) in cultured endothelial cells and in atherosclerosis-prone areas of hypercholesterolemic mice. Moreover, oral administration of pomegranate juice to hypercholesterolemic mice at various stages of the disease, significantly reduced the progression of atherosclerosis. This experimental study indicates that the proatherogenic effects induced by perturbed shear stress can be reversed by chronic administration of pomegranate juice.

Watermelon and nitric oxide

July 11, 2008, Greencastle, Indiana, new research suggests that consuming watermelon rinds -- which contain the amino acid citrulline -- could play a role in relaxing blood vessels and creating
160

what is known as a "Viagra effect." The work shows that the body converts citrulline to arginine, which in turn boosts nitric oxide. The work was conducted at Texas A&M University.

An article in New Mexico's Las Cruces Sun-News notes, "Dr. Ferid Murad, who shared a Nobel Prize in 1998 for his research on nitric oxide, including identifying its role in nitroglycerin, told the Washington Post in 2003 that citrulline 'acts only marginally in recycling L-arginine' to increase nitric oxide." Murad is a 1958 graduate of DePauw University.

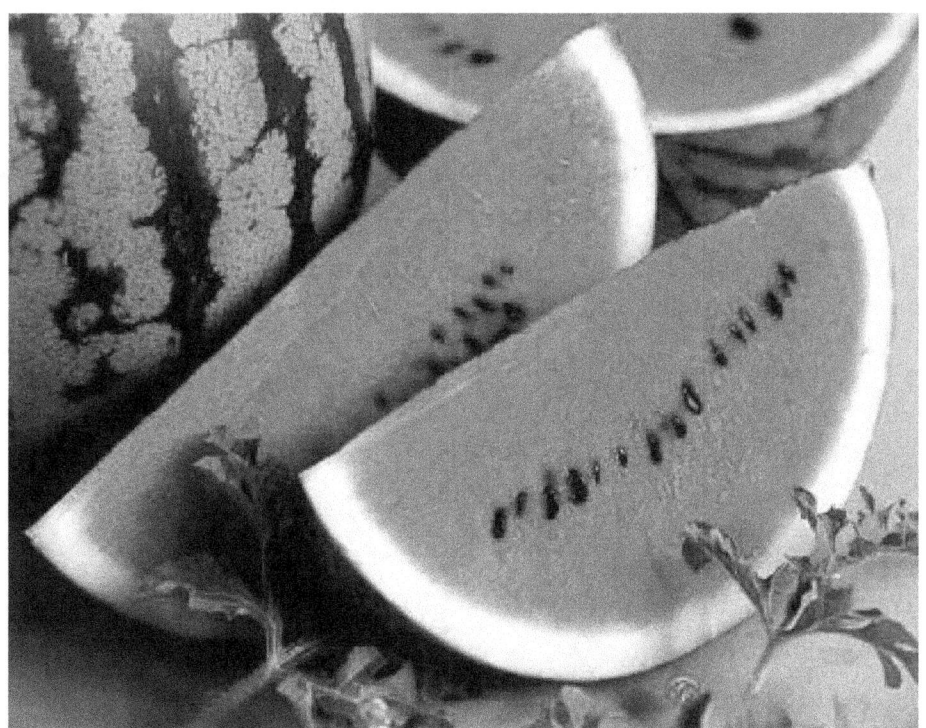

TCM and nitric oxide

Dr. Murad knew about TCMs long ago, He said

"It's not really a new territory, but the idea came from my work with nitric oxide. About 20 years ago, I was the vice president of pharmaceutical research and development in Abbott Laboratory. It's a bigmultina tional company and I was in charge of all the clinical pharmaceutical research and basic research to discover drugs, and I was asked by my superior, what do we do with our natural products program? We had a small natural products program working with herbal extracts. Do we improve the program or do we get rid of it?

I just joined the company and I knew a little bit about TCMs, because I used to be an editor for the book--Goodman & Gilman's The Pharmacological Basis of Therapeutics, really a famous pharmacology book. And we talk a lot about TCMs' historical use and how they work, I knew some of the TCMs, e.g. reserpine to treat hypertension. I knew about salicylate extracts from tree bark work, taxol came from an extract for cancer treatment. The statins also came from the extracts for cholesterol treatment. So there are examples that the TCMs resulted in important western drugs.

And, as I began thinking about TCM extracts, I became more and more intrigued as I knew more and more about nitric oxide biology and biochemistry. I knew about that the cofactors to support the activity of the nitric oxide enzymes, or influenced their oxidation state. All these drugs enhance cyclic GMP and / or cyclic AMP production.

And I said to myself, perhaps the TCMs are antioxidants. They might be regulation of cyclic GMP or cyclic AMP. I wanted to study some TCMs to see if they work on nitric oxide.

And I was able to get the Shanghai University of TCMs in Shanghai, to give me research lab space, some money and equipment to study this. It has been 7 years since I have studied TCM extracts. 100 extracts we've tested. We find them by looking at the literature. Do these extracts effect stroke, hypertension, heart attack and the things I know nitric oxide may be have effects? So we took those 100 extracts and screened them. We have about 20 that we think may work through nitric oxide. Now I think that's the important first step, because by knowing that they work through nitric oxide we are going to figure out how they work. Do they enhance the formation nitric oxide, do they increase the activity of NOS. What enzymes do they affect? And by knowing that, we are going be able to use some of the TCMs for other diseases. We also are going to take these extracts and put them together to make them even more effective.

Someday we'll be able to identify the active ingredients in the extracts to make western drugs. So it's been a fun project. I think we are making progress."

Establish correct health-care concept

It is widely assumed that health-care products are only effective if the effects of the supplements can be observed within a short period of time. In fact this is not the case.

As a nutritional supplement, health-care products only compensate the inadequacy of certain nutrients required by the human body in our daily diet. However, all the nutrients are metabolized in the human body, which is unable to synthesize many nutrients by itself. Therefore, it is necessary to take these nutritional supplements regularly, just as we would eat meals and drink water every day.

In USA, the annual sales of nutritional supplements amount to $50 billion and daily intake of different necessary supplements has become a necessary daily practice. This indicates not only a high awareness about healthcare but also a widespread understanding of what is crucial to human health.

In fact health-care is a long-term undertaking and it is neither realistic nor scientific to think that such problems can be solved immediately. Only if nutrients are ingested over a long period of time can they be effective and their effects be felt in the body.

How to correctly choose nitric oxide dietary supplement

1.Choose products made by world renowned scientific research team and avoid using products without proper scientific theory.

2.Choose products made from world cutting-edge biomedical technology and avoid products that might content toxic substance or might cause side-effect.

3.Choose products made from natural ingredient.

4.Choose products that can stably release nitric oxide and avoid taking product that causes nitric oxide level in the body to rise suddenly, which will cause stress to cardio-vascular system.

5.Choose products that the effectiveness has been proved by human trial, products which are backed up by realistic data.

6.Choose products which are being sold by large scale cooperation with excellent background.

7.Choose products that have been on the market for a period of time and well reputed from the customers.

Chapter Four
Antioxidant Supplements

Aging in the human body is in fact a slow process of oxidation, which accelerates over time. Therefore, it is essential to take anti-oxidation functional food supplements to prevent the oxidation of cells and prolong good health and life span.

Antioxidants, which may be found in certain foodstuffs or health-care products, can increase the NO level in the human body by clearing or neutralizing harmful free radicals. Such free radicals are produced in the process of in vivo oxidative stress. By removing free radicals, antioxidants can repair vascular endothelial cells that generate nitric oxide, and prevent inadequate nitric oxide generation. It is therefore important to understand: which diseases are related to nitric oxide deficiency? What kind of functional foods should be supplemented to improve such diseases?

Cancer (Top of Ten Major Causes of death in the World)

Useful antioxidant functional foods:
1) Compound vitamins (Vitamin A, Vitamin C, Vitamin E, B Vitamins, folic acid, etc)
Vitamins are effective antioxidants, which can clear in vivo free radicals and avoid oxidation related cell injury. Additionally, folic acid has also proven effective at combating cancer. If the human body is short of folic acid, chromosomes of cellular tissues will become weak, and may be easily injured by oxidation.
2) Soybean isoflavone

Soybean isoflavone extracted from soybeans is a kind of estrogen similar to the female hormone. Its most basic component, "genistein" is extremely effective at inhibiting the growth of tumor cells (especially those that cause breast cancer and prostate cancer).

3) Shark cartilage

Shark cartilage comprises various mucopolysaccharide proteins and its primary component "chondroitin" is one of the most physiologically active components in shark cartilage. Being different from protein, in addition to enhancement of immune capacity, mucopolysaccharide in chondroitin is also taken as natural anti-inflammation and wound-curing treatment. Chondroitin is noted for its anti-angiogenic factor, which can stop the generation of cancer cells. As the growth and spread of cancer cells is a result of the angiogenic effect, shark cartilage is an essential functional food for cancer patients.

4) Lycopene

As a member of the β-carotene group, lycopene has 11 consecutive conjugated double bonds of carotenoid, which give it an excellent capacity to remove free radicals. The efficacy of lycopene in

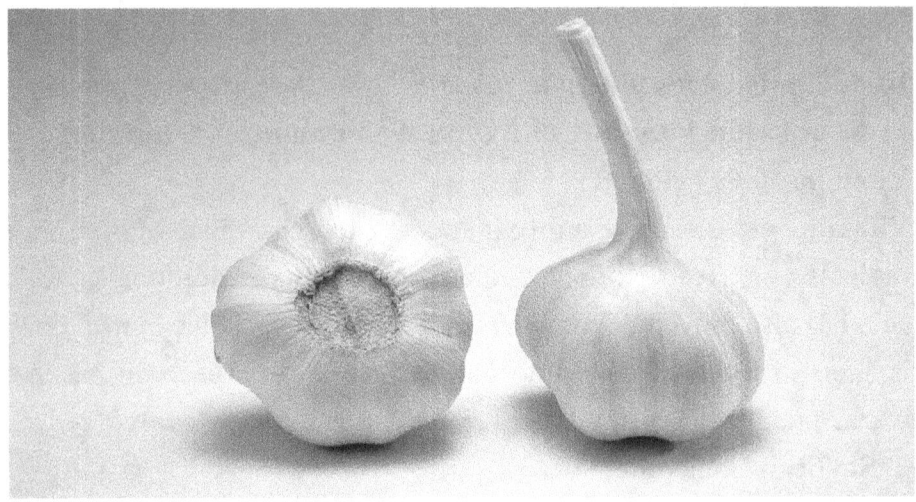

inhibiting cancer cells is 33 times that of carotene, and is highly effective at preventing bladder cancer, pancreatic cancer, skin cancer, breast cancer, prostate cancer, lung cancer, oral cancer, gastric cancer, and ovarian cancer.

5) Garlic

Garlic is considered one of the most valuable foods on the earth. Its major active component is allicin, also known as the "natural antibiotic". Garlic is used in a variety of applications. As research by the US National Cancer Institute (NCI) shows, regular consumption of garlic can reduce the risk of esophagus cancer, gastric cancer and colon cancer. This is because garlic can increase the activity of leukocytes and phagocytes, promote human immunity and reduce the formation of carcinogenic substances. What is more, garlic is also able to reduce blood pressure. Since ancient times, it has always been one of the most popular functional foods.

6) Coenzyme Q_{10}

Coenzyme Q_{10} is a kind of co-ferment, also known as "ubiquinone". It is fat-soluble diphenol, with a structure similar to Vitamin K. Since Coenzyme Q_{10} shows a special efficacy in cardiomyopathy, it is also called the "heart-care element" or "heart-care enzyme".

Coenzyme Q_{10} can help cells transform nutrients into ATP. It is an indispensable substance for energy production within cells.

Coenzyme Q_{10} can help maintain the integrity of DNA and membranes.

Coenzyme Q_{10} is a very strong antioxidant, and its anti-cancer effect has been proven by many medical studies. According to a report by American Dr. Karl Folkers, when Coenzyme Q_{10} was used to treat 10 cancer patients, 6 of the patients made a full recovery. Danish Dr.

Knut Lockwood also used different antioxidants, including Coenzyme Q_{10} for treating breast cancer patients, with highly successful results. It should be noted, however, that they all took Coenzyme Q_{10} as auxiliaries for treatment.

Hypertension, cerebrovascular and cardiovascular diseases

Useful antioxidant functional foods:
1) Ginkgo extract
Ginkgo is a powerful antioxidant, with the main function of preventing free radicals from damaging the brain and neurons and strengthening the conductive and sensing functions of the nervous system. It can also prevent cerebral cell disorder and vessel congestion in the heart and limbs. It is an ideal health-care product for prevention and treatment of cerebral and cardiovascular diseases.
2) Coenzyme Q_{10}
Coenzyme Q_{10} is currently the most popular heart protector, known as "heart-care element". It can prevent hypertension, enhance myocardium, and repair heart injuries and other muscle tissues, as well as being an effective treatment for cerebral and cardiovascular diseases.
3) Deep-sea king fish oil
Deep-sea king fish oil contains the rare Omega-3 unsaturated fatty acid, including EPA (eicosapentaenoic acid) and DHA (docosahexaenoic acid). The fish oil has been recognized as useful for improving heart function, reducing hypertension, and preventing cardiovascular diseases. Omega-3 is essential to the human body, and cannot independently be synthesized in the body. It has been shown to help lower cholesterol, hypertension and reduce the incidence

of cardiomyopathy and strokes. EPA and DHA are both capable of increasing the activation of cerebral cells and promoting memory and learning capacity. DHA is a very important nutrient for the growth and development of infants and young children.

4) Lecithin

Lecithin extracted from soybeans can enhance cerebral cells and normalize the neurotransmission of information and transport function. Lecithin is also a kind of emulsifier, and can help cholesterol fat to combine with protein, for transmission, via blood, to different tissue cells.

5) Garlic extract

Garlic contains multiple sulfides, amino acid, minerals and cellulose. The effects of sulfide include reducing and decreasing blood clots, cholesterol and triglyceride. It can also inhibit the growth of microbes and protect cardiac vessels as well as preventing strokes.

6) Evening primrose oil

Evening primrose has been used since ancient times and has been honored in China as the "universal medicine for emperors". The oil extracted from its seeds contains special multi-element unsaturated fatty acids, about 70% of which is gamma-linolenic acid and about 10% of which is γ-linseed oil fatty acid. Neither of them can be independently synthesized by the human body. Many studies have proven that it can help prevent atherosclerosis and hypertension, lower cholesterol and reduce the incidence of cardiovascular diseases. It is also highly effective at preventing diabetes and helping to treat hepatic cirrhosis.

Erectile dysfunction

Useful antioxidant functional foods:

1) Herba epimedii

Herba epimedii contains icariin and cpimedoside, both of which have the effect of enhancing sexual desire. The mechanism is: after semen is secreted and the hyperfunction and seminal vesicle is filled, the sensory nerve is stimulated to trigger sexual arousal indirectly.

2) Maca

Maca contains a huge amount of protein, mineral zinc, taurine and other components. The rich amino acids found in protein alone are necessary for maintaining the health of the human body. Such components are effective at helping the body to resist fatigue. Maca can improve sexual function, increase sperm count, promote the vitality of sperm, and effectively improve sexual function by regulating the endocrine system and hormone balance.

3) Herba cistanche

Cistanche is honored as "desert ginseng". It contains significant quantities of amino acid, cystine, vitamins, minerals and other rare nutritional components, and has a great invigorating effect on such organs as the male kidney, testis, penis, and cavernosum. It is also excellent at preventing impotence and premature ejaculation.

Immune deficiency

Useful antioxidant functional foods:
1) Astragalus
Astragalus contains flavonoid and saponin, both of which have

170

relatively high antioxidative effects and are therefore able to remove in vivo free radicals. By regulating the density of free calcium in spleen lymphocytes and promoting cellular protein kinase activity, astragalus polysaccharide contained in astragalus can affect the signal of organic immune cells, thereby enhancing immune regulation.

2) Chinese dates

Jujube polysaccharide, is an active substance in Chinese dates that promotes proliferation of lymphocytes. It can improve body immunity. Additionally, Vitamin C found in Chinese dates is an antioxidant and can effectively remove in vivo oxygen free radicals and protect cells against oxidative injury.

3) Cornus officinalis

Cornel polysaccharide, which is found in cornus officinalis has the effect of enhancing immunity. Cornel polysaccharide can also significantly increase the phagocytic index of mouse peritoneal macrophages and promote the formation of hemolysin and the transformation of lymphocytes.

4) American ginseng

As the first choice of medical material for invigoration and health care, American ginseng (panax) contains panax polysaccharide and panaquilon and can help strengthen the immune system. By promoting synthesis of serum proteins, marrow proteins and organic proteins, the components can improve body immunity and effectively resist cancer by inhibiting the growth of cancer cells.

5) Green tea

Green tea can reduce fatigue, and has powerful anti-oxidizing and relaxing effects. Green tea also contains Vitamin C and flavonoids, which enhance the antioxidative efficacy of Vitamin C. These flavonoids are also valuable nutritional products and can keep skin healthy.

Lung diseases

Useful antioxidant functional foods:
1) Vitamin A, Vitamin C, B Vitamins
Vitamin A is an element necessary for maintaining mucosa in the respiratory tract. Lack of Vitamin A will increase the probability of respiratory tract infection and increases the probability of pneumonia. Vitamin C is an important antioxidative food for resisting viruses and inflammation and is highly beneficial to the lungs. The Vitamin B group can enhance physical strength, contribute to the production of antibodies, is necessary for the formation of erythrocytes, strengthens the immune system, and reduces the likelihood of contracting pneumonia.

2) Garlic
The antibiotic function of garlic is well known. It contains sulfide that is highly effective at inhibiting microbes, bacteria and fungi as well as strengthening immunity and effectively reducing the formation of pneumonia.

3) Echinacea extract
Echinacea is capable of preventing inflammation, resisting bacterial infection and helping in excretion of toxins. In particular, it can promote a rapid increase in the effectiveness of the immune system. As early as in the 19 century, it was used as a medicinal herb and was thought to be capable of treating almost all infectious diseases. It has more than 70 effective components, the main ones of which are: polysaccharides, flavonoids, endothelin, Vitamin A, Vitamin C, Vitamin E, potassium, sulfur, iodine, iron, copper and minerals.

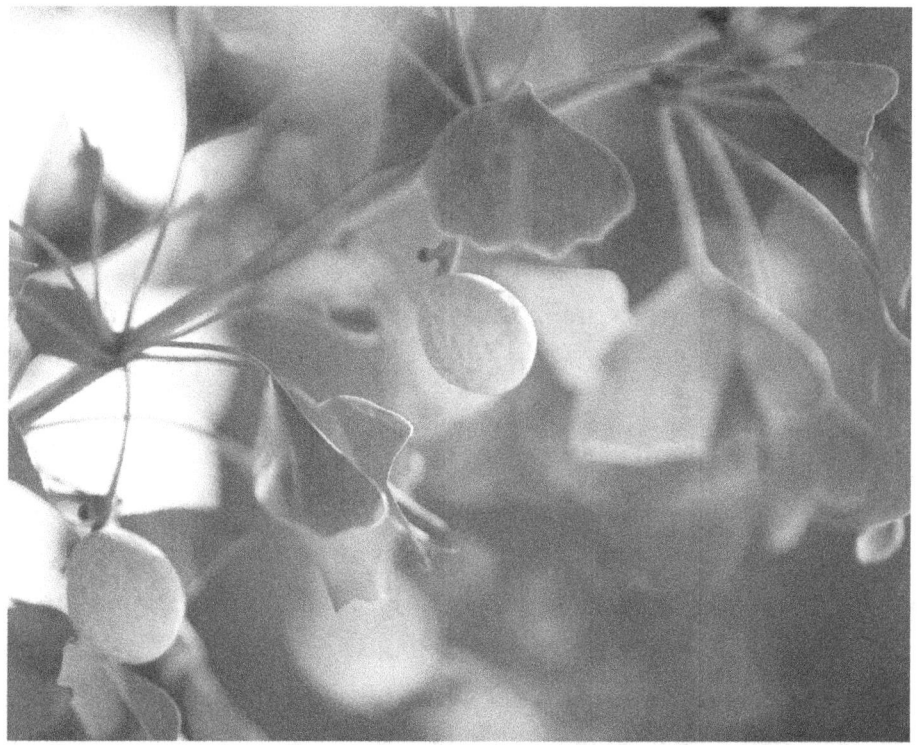

Echinacea can be combined with other foodstuffs effectively to become one of the most ideal stimuli to the immune system.

4) Ginkgo

Since ancient times, the Chinese have been aware of the many benefits of ginkgo. Ginkgo can benefit the brain, nourish the heart and is an effective treatment for eczema. Ginkgo is also capable of treating diseases related to blood circulation and respiratory tract disorders such as coughing. The ancient Indian physician Ayuveda considered the use of gingko to be the key to longevity. Nowadays, gingko is in high demand as a functional food throughout the developed world.

Liver diseases

Useful antioxidant functional foods:
1) Vitamin A, Vitamin C, Vitamin E and B Vitamins
Vitamin A, Vitamin C, Vitamin E and B Vitamins are all antioxidants. B Vitamins are indirect antioxidants. They help maintain normal metabolism in the liver and mitigate fatigue due to injury to the liver, and are the first defense for liver protection and maintenance.

2) Milk thistle extract
The silymarin in milk thistle extract helps to enhance the functions of the liver, decompose fat and repair and maintain liver tissues. Additionally, it is able to promote protein synthesis in hepatocyte cells, promote hepatocyte production, enhance the antioxidative capacity of hepatocytes, and repel invading toxins. Due to its therapeutic function for different liver diseases, milk thistle extract has been highly praised in medical circles.

3) Lecithin
Lecithin is extracted from soybeans and has the function of removing fat as well as preventing "fatty liver". It can also delay the aging of the liver and is capable of repairing and caring for the liver when it is damaged by alcohol. What is more, since lecithin can also lubricate the intestinal tract and soften feces, it can be used to treat constipation and prevent toxins and free radicals from injuring the liver.

4) Garlic
Sulfide in garlic can remove toxins from the blood and liver, and can be used to prevent and treat liver diseases that occur as a result of exposure to air pollution.

Renal diseases

Useful antioxidant functional foods:

1) Vitamin C and B Vitamins

Vitamin C has the effect of acidifying urine for antibacterial purposes as well as improving the function of the immune system. Vitamin B_6 is beneficial for eliminating edema and increasing renal function.

2) Cranberry extract

Cranberry extract containing procyanidine is an excellent natural antibiotic. In addition to its role as a highly effective treatment for urethra infections and cystitis, it can also be used to treat urinary incontinence and kidney stones. Furthermore, the antioxidative effect of cranberry extract may promote human immunity and is useful for prevention and treatment of renal diseases.

3) Lecithin

Lecithin is rich in insoitol and choline and is useful for patients suffering from renal diseases. In addition, lecithin can also enhance the capacity of bile to dissolve cholesterol and prevent cholelithiasis.

Diabetes

Useful antioxidant functional foods:

1) Vitamin C, Vitamin E, β- carotene

The blood glucose value of diabetic patients is higher than normal, indicating a poor metabolism. Similarly, the concentration of in vivo cause of damage to the pancreas and related complications. Therefore, ingesting more antioxidants, such as Vitamin C and Vitamin E is helpful for stabilizing the physical condition of those suffering from diabetes.

2) Ginkgo extract

Ginkgo can mitigate worsening diabetes and reduce the incidence of complications, such as retinal lesions, peripheral nerve necrosis, amputation, renal failure and uremia. This is because the flavonoid in ginkgo has a protective effect against hypoxia of neurons that occurs due to diabetes or poor blood circulation. It is also capable of increasing the utilization rate of glucose by cells and promoting the sensitivity of cells to insulin.

3) Ginseng

Since the ancient times, ginseng has been one of the most valuable medicinal substances used in China. It is capable of supplementing physical strength and energy and promoting sexual capability. In China, it is known as "king of invigorators", and is also closely linked to longevity. Ginseng contains Vitamin B_1, B_2, B_6 and B_{12}, biotin, choline, minerals, saccharine, flavonoids and ginseng saponin. Ginseng saponin can prevent and treat various chronic diseases including diabetes as it is capable of stabilizing the value of blood glucose.

4) Cranberry extract

One of the most severe complications of diabetes is ocular retinal lesions. Procyanidine, which is found in cranberries is highly effective at promoting ocular vascular circulation for protecting the eyes and is useful for diabetic patients.

5) Beer yeast

Beer yeast contains various nutrients essential for the human body, including protein (which comprises 50% of the overall nutritional content), B Vitamins, 16 types of amino acids, 17 types of Vitamins, natural cellulose, and 14 types of minerals including chromium, selenium and iron. It should also be noted that beer yeast is rich in trace elements such as chromium. Chromium can control the glucose content of blood and keep blood stable for relatively long periods of time. In the USA, new medical studies suggest that chromium can improve the condition of non-insulin dependent Type-II diabetes patients. Many doctors that specialize in metabolism recommend that patients increase their chromium intake, making beer yeast a very good choice as a nutritional supplement.

Gastrointestinal tract diseases

Useful antioxidant functional foods:
1) Vitamin A, Vitamin C, Vitamin E, B Vitamins (compound vitamins) and minerals

B Vitamins can enhance stomach and intestine functions; Vitamin E can reduce gastric acid levels and reduce pain; Vitamin A and Vitamin C help to protect the mucosa and enhance injury recovery; zinc can mitigate ulcers; iron can prevent anemia and hemorrhagic ulcers.

2) Aloe extract

Aloe contains mucopolysaccharide and has an excellent protective effect on the gastrointestinal tract mucosa. It can mitigate the secretion of gastric acid and increase the recovery of gastriointestinal mucosa cells and tissues. In addition to enhancing gastrointestinal functions, aloe is also capable of mitigating the effects of pain and ulcers in the body.

3) Garlic

The allicin and sulfide present in garlic both have strong antibacterial effects and can inhibit the growth of gastric ulcer bacteria. If garlic is used in combination with chemical substances that can reduce gastric acid, the effect will be enhanced even further. In addition, garlic is also helpful for digestion and is beneficial for treatment of digestive ulcer diseases.

4) Cranberry extract

The active substances present in cranberry are highly efficient at removing urinary tract bacteria, and treating microbe infections. According to the latest research, special compounds in cranberry can also inhibit helicobacter pylori effectively. Bacteria such as these are the main cause for gastric digestive ulcers and cranberries are able to treat ulcers by inhibiting the adhesion of bacteria to the endothelia cells of the gastric mucosa.

Constipation

Useful antioxidant functional foods:
1) Vitamin A, Vitamin C, Vitamin E, and B Vitamins (compound vitamins)

B Vitamins can help in the digestion of fat and saccharide proteins and are therefore effective treatments for the symptoms of constipation, especially Vitamins B_1, B_2, and B_{12} as well as folic acid, nicotinic acid and pantothen.

2) Aloe extract

The unique components contained in aloe are emodin. aloe-emodin and aloin. These have the effect of resisting bacteria and promoting colorectal evacuation as well as cleansing the intestines and softening feces.

3) Beer yeast

The B Vitamins present in beer yeast can treat constipation as well as maintain the balance of useful enteral bacteria. Furthermore, beer yeast contains significant quantities of cellulose, which can promote enterogastric peristalsis, which shortens the time for food to pass through the small intestines.

4) Lecithin

Lecithin is a well-known emulsifier that can promote the digestion and absorption of fat and fat-soluble vitamins as well as promote the propagation of healthy bacteria in the intestine. As it is hydrophilic, lecithin can help maintain the water content of the intestinal tract, which lubricates the intestinal tract, and softens feces.

Premenstrual complications

Useful antioxidant functional foods:
1) Compound vitamins and minerals

Vitamin B_6 can alleviate water retention, mammary swelling pains, emotional instability, and fatigue; Vitamin B_1 and B_2 can effectively reduce premenstrual waist and foot aches, abdominal distension and

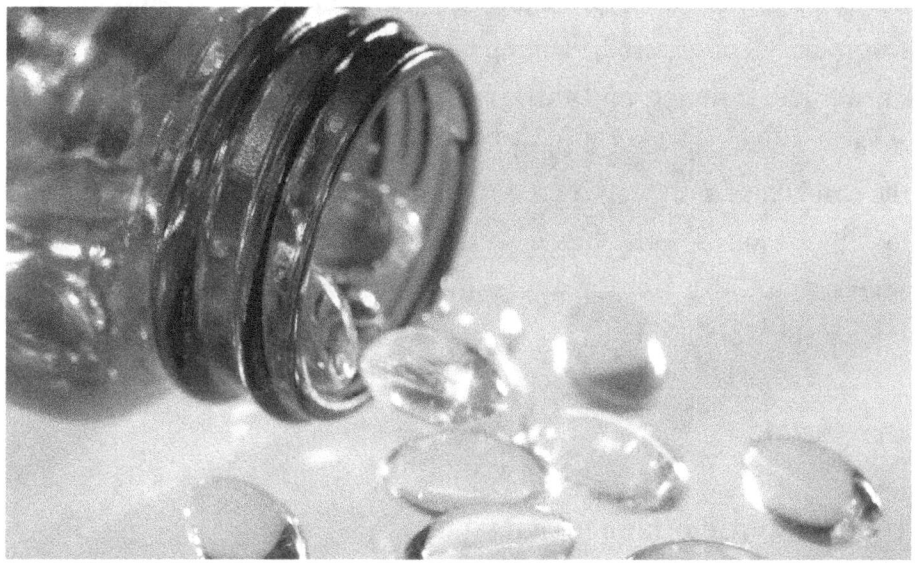

pain, and prevent oral ulcers. Folic acid and Vitamin B_{12} are "blood-making vitamins", which can prevent anemia Vitamin Cand Vitamin E are antioxidants that can mitigate such symptoms as emotional anxiety, depression and premenstrual swelling; Vitamin A and Vitamin D are also helpful in mitigating premenstrual depression and excessive secretion of skin oil. As for minerals, magnesium can treat emotional discomfort due to cervicodynia, tinnitus and abdominal pain, while iron can enrich the blood, while calcium is also able to mitigate menstrual discomfort. Magnesium can also help cardiovascular disorders.

2) Deep-sea king fish oil

In deep-sea king fish oil, omega-3 polyunsaturated fatty acid, DHA and EPA, are very helpful in balancing female hormones. EPA and DHA are also useful for treating female physiological symptoms, and decreasing cholesterol.

3) Evening primrose oil

Evening primrose is rich in gamma-linolenic acid (GLA), which is also categorized as an omega-6 polyunsaturated fatty acid (similar to omega-3 contained in deep-sea king fish oil). It can regulate hormones, balance and mitigate uterine contraction, and relieve menstruation pain and discomfort. In addition, it can help maintain the cell health and treat rough skin during menstruation. In addition to evening primrose oil, borage seed, ligustrum lucidum ait and fructus lycii oil are also rich in γ- gamma-linolenic acid and are all well-known for women.

Depression

Useful antioxidant functional foods:

180

1) Compound vitamins

Many vitamins produce the effect of resisting depression. For instance, B Vitamins are a widely known treatment for depression, with the most effective of which are Vitamin B_1, B_6 and B_{12}. Lack of folic acid will result in symptoms of psychosis and easily lead to such phenomena as low mood. Free radicals are a major enemy of the human body and may easily injure neurons in the human body. According to the latest research, antioxidant supplements such as Vitamins C and E can also prevent and treat depression.

2) Deep-sea king fish oil

Its omega-3 polyunsaturated fatty acid has an effect similar to antidepression drugs: block neural conduction route, increase the secretion of serotonin, and reduce melancholia.

3) St. John's wort

St. John's wort (Chinese hericium) was used in Europe as an anti-septic in the past. However, according to recent studies, its biggest advantage may be its function as a treatment for depression. St. John's wort extract contains more than 10 biologically active ingredients, of which hypericin has the effect of calming the emotions. It will increase the concentration of the in vivo neural transmitter serotonin in blood. Serotonin, which is associated with sleeping, mood, prolactin secretion and can produce an effect similar to that of Prozac, but without almost any side effects.

4) Valerian

Valerian is famously effective at stabilizing nerves, relaxing the central nervous system and reducing muscle pain and muscle soreness. Since ancient times, it has been considered an effective medicine used for stabilizing the nerves and promoting regular sleeping patterns. It can also be used to relieve melancholy, and can reduce the neural transmitter activity of the intracerebral excitatory nervous system, allowing patients to become calm and relieve feelings of tension, anxiety and depression.

Senile dementia

Useful antioxidant functional foods:
1) Compound vitamins
All vitamins are critical to controlling the onset of senile dementia. For instance , Vitamin A, Vitamin C, and Vitamin E are all antioxidants, which can reduce injury to cerebral cells from free radicals; Vitamin B_{12} and folic acid have been linked to neural development and are capable of keeping the nervous system healthy.
2) Ginkgo extract
Ginkgo is highly effective at enhancing memory function and can promote systemic blood circulation, especially cerebral blood circulation.
3) Ginseng
Ginseng is an excellent anti-aging substance, as well as being nourishing and refreshing. For this reason it enjoys a reputation as one of the best nutritional supplements for the elderly. Ginseng saponin displays a highly beneficial pharmacological effect on the central nerves, endocrine system, and cardiovascular system. According to recent research, the major active component of ginseng, ginsengsaponin is extremely effective at stimulating mental activity. It is especially useful for maintaining cognitive functions such as learning capacity and memory among elderly individuals.
4) Lecithin
Lecithin is an important component of synthetic neural conductors

and is very useful for enhancing memory and attention span, as well as preventing senile dementia.

5) Deep-sea king fish oil

The EPA and DHA contained in deep-sea king fish oil can decrease cholesterol and prevent cardiovascular diseases. DHA is an essential nutrient for cerebral and retinal development, and is highly effective at preventing memory failure and senile dementia.

Rheumatism, arthritis, gout

Useful antioxidant functional foods:
1) Compound vitamins and minerals

In vivo free radicals are one of the major causes of arthritis, gout and rheumatism. Use of antioxidants can alleviate the effects of arthritis, rheumatism and gout. Vitamin C and Vitamin E are both very good antioxidants. For patients suffering from gout, it must be noted that excessive Vitamin A, Vitamin C and nicotinic acid may stimulate the formation of uric acid. B Vitamins and folic acid can prevent the level of uric acid in blood from rising, and are important substances for treating gout.

Calcium, magnesium, selenium and zinc are all essential elements, and are very useful for prevention and treatment of arthritis.

2) Evening primrose oil

Both evening primrose oil and borage seed oil are rich in gamma-linolenic acid, which, in addition to their usefulness towards alleviating the effects of menstruation are effective treatments for arthritic pain, especially for rheumatic arthritis.

3) Glucosamine chondroitin

This can help injured cartilage, promote the metabolism of cartilage and prevent joint inflammation, as well as having the effect of decreasing pain. It also helps cartilage to absorb nutrition so that it becomes more elastic. It is the best nutritional supplement for treating degenerative arthritis.

4) Celery seed

In traditional therapies, celery seed is used to handle different types of arthritis. Celery seed contains more than twenty types of anti-inflammatory components and promotes in vitro elimination of uric acid. It is a form of natural diuretic as well as a good therapy for gout and arthritis.

Any of the above antioxidant functional foods can be combined with other antioxidants such as grape seeds to create an even stronger complementary effect.

Retinal lesions

Useful antioxidant functional foods:
1) Lutein

Human eyes are rich in lutein, which is the main pigment in the human ocular retinal macular area. This element cannot be synthesized by the human body and must be supplemented.

Upon entering the eyes, blue light from the sunlight spectrum may run directly through the eyeball to reach the retinal macula, while at the same time producing a significant quantity of free radicals. Lutein is known as "adelomorphic sunglasses". As a pigment, the lutein in the macula can filter out the blue light and, as an antioxidant, can remove free radicals, thereby preventing the outer layer of fat in the macular area from suffering oxidative injury of free radicals.

2) Extracts of blueberry, cowberry and grape rich in anthocyanin

Anthocyanin can improve the microcirculation of the human body, enhance the supply of nutrition to the retina, improve retinal function, and increase sensitivity.

Additionally, around the human eyeground veins, there is a high-density antioxidant, but as the human body ages, the antioxidative protection effect in the human body will be gradually decreased, and the effect of anthocyanin in removing in vivo free radicals assumes considerable importance.

Chapter Five
The Physiotherapy of Nitric Oxide - Laughter

Laughter is the most moving expression of interpersonal communication. It is a beautiful and silent language in social life. Laughter comes from an origin of kindness, tolerance and selflessness of one's heart. It shows how straightforward and magnanimous a person is. Laughter connects people, and it is also beneficial to a person's health.

Laughter has the following regulation function to the human body:

1.Regulates muscle system

Laughter can drive the chest, abdomen, back of the waist, lips and facial muscle movement at the same time. In the time of laughter, a total of 80 muscles of the whole body are in motion. The motion of laughter allows the contraction of thirteen facial muscles; these muscles are then allowed to relax after the contraction.

A study found that abdominally driven laughter is equivalent to 10 minutes of exercise on the treadmill. It works out all of the main muscle regions of the whole body. Therefore, laughter is said to be equivalent to an "internal jogging". Although cachinnation can increase blood pressure and heart rate, however, after laughing, blood pressure and heart rate will decrease to lower than normal level. It can almost achieve the effect of exercising. For the old and the sick that have difficulty to participate in exercises, laughter will benefit them as an alternative way to exercise.

2. Protects cardiovascular system

Happy laughter can provide a good amount of blood flow to the heart and reduces blood pressure. It improves circulation throughout the

186

whole body as well as local microcirculation.

In a recent study conducted by the Maryland University, it is found that when people laugh, vascular endothelial expands and releases nitric oxide. It reduces possibility of blood clotting and better prevents pathogen infection. It helps to regulate blood circulation, improves cardiovascular function and subsequently reducing the risk of heart disease.

The latest research shows that a jovial laughter, not only can regulate human body's blood pressure and vascular tone, it also can stimulate hypothalamus pituitary gland to secrete endorphins and opioid. Then, through the activation of μ - opioid receptor, the expression in endothelial up-regulates nitric oxide synthase and enhances the production of nitric oxide. Nitric oxide exerts a variety of cardio-protective cellular processes via cellular signaling pathways. It includes a cGMP-dependent pathway responsible for vasodilation, reducing platelet aggregation as well as inhibition of leucocytes trafficking for the reduction of vascular inflammation.

Laughter can function as a useful and important tactic to promote cardiovascular health.

By laughing every day, it lowers c-reactive protein level in the body and high c-reactive protein level is associated with heart attack.

For diabetes patients who are at high risk of multiple heart diseases, laughing also reduces their risk of getting such complications.

Maintaining a happy mood also helps to regulate blood glucose level.

For diabetic patients, happy mood can benignly stimulate the brain, and causes the secretion of the hormone that excites the circulation of the cardiovascular system. It promotes the level of the so-called "good cholesterol", high-density lipoprotein, to rise. It in turns promotes the health of the cardiovascular system.

A scientific research team in the University of Loma Linda California selected twenty 50 year old in average patients with type II diabetes and divided them into two groups. They all had hypertension and had high cholesterol level; they were at high risk of heart attack. After one year of study, data showed that for the group of patients that watched comedy movies and laughed every day, the "good cholesterol" level in the body rose by 26%. In the control group patients, the level only rose 3%. The "good cholesterol" level in the cardiovascular system has protective effect, and aids to reduce the risk of heart attack.

2.Regulating the autonomic nervous system

Laughter can balance the autonomic nervous system and regulate hormone secretion and the immune system. It allows the body and mind to relax, in turn fine-tunes the neuroendocrine system.

A large number of studies showed that laughter can promote the secretion of endorphins. Endorphin is a chemical substance that exists in the brain and the nervous tissue, which possesses euphoria effect similar to morphine analgesia. For people who suffer from spondylitis, arthritis and muscle spasm, laughter helps to alleviate pain. Laughter has easing effect to migraine and tension headache, it can even help to reduce postoperative pain, and relieving nervousness.

4. Promotes digestion, regulates immune functions

Laughter can increase appetite, increase the level of digestive juice and promote the secretion of digestive enzymes; which promotes digestion of food and absorption of nutrients. Laughter also helps to increase the number of immune cells and boost the immune system.

A study found that, when the patient receives "humor therapy" with laughing and mood relaxation treatment, it increases the lymph cell by 10% to 14%, which acts positively on the body's immune function.

5. Relieves stress

Laughter expresses feelings healthily and helps to relieve mental conflicts. Genuine laughter can dispel distress of the spirits and helps to overcome shyness, embarrassment and various kinds of troubles; it improves mental health significantly.

6. Communicates harmoniously

Laughter is a type of genuine facial expression that shortens the psychological distance between persons, bridges interpersonal relationships and makes communication easier. Laughter generates warm and friendly atmosphere, it is the best interpersonal lubricant.

7. Beautifying effect

Smiling action often exercise the facial muscle elasticity, prevents from skin laxity and wrinkling. It also warms skin tone and improves complexity due to the accelerated facial microcirculation.

8. How to induce healthy laughs

Watch comedy

Watching the comedian's exaggerated expression and funny storyline and have a good laugh. A good laugh repels heavy mood, this works better than any drugs.

Spend more time with happy people

Happy mood is transmissible. By being with happy people, one is more prone to be in a happier mood as well.

Smile to the mirror everyday

A mirror is the best tool to practice smiling or laughing with. It is healthy to practice laughing in the mirror every day, several times regularly.

The world will be a much more beautiful place if we all laugh more every day. Laughter is the best health supplement; it is one of the secrets to longevity. If you want to live harmoniously, please laugh. If you want to be a happier person, please laugh. Laughter is always your best friend, forever!

Chapter Six
The Physiotherapy of Nitric Oxide – Vibration Bed

One: The harmfulness of sub-health status of human body

In recent years, as modern social life advances, the rhythm of lifestyle speeds up day by day. Competitive nature in work force creates immense amount of pressure in working adults.

A large population is constantly under physical and mental stress, such population includes: the working crowd, especially the highly-stressed white-collar workers, the frequent travelling businessmen, the over-trained athletes and students who are under immense stress from exam preparation; they are all physically deteriorated, energy strained with chances of developing chronic diseases. They are in the dangerous zone between healthiness and illness. This grey area is defined as the "third state" - the state of sub-health.

The status of being in the "sub-health" state has becoming a serious health problem among most people.

According to the latest research, being in the sub-health status bears five big hazards:

1) The sub-health status is the status before the development of most non-communicable chronic diseases

2) The sub-health status affects work, life and learning ability significantly

3) Could cause possible mental disorders

4) Affects sleep, aggravating physical and mental fatigue

5) Affects lifespan

The sub-health status can evolve into two different results: one is through effective conditioning; it can transition back to a healthy state. The other less desired result is that, if ignored, the health state might slowly deteriorate and progresses towards the direction of disease formation. It is also possible for the incident of "karoshi" (occupational sudden death) to occur. Therefore, it is a crucial mission for people to avoid being in this "sub-health" health state.

The best way to avoid this sub-health condition is to change one's psychological and physical behavior altogether. Having the right health knowledge, being in a healthy diet, having healthy lifestyles, getting the right amount of exercise, avoid smoking and excessive alcohol consumption, being in a healthy mental state, etc; these are all essential practices for living healthfully.

Two: Physical therapy and nitric oxide

Physiotherapy is a type of treatment effectively utilizing natural or artificial physical forces on the human body in the intention of disease treatment or prevention. Physiotherapy is an important division in modern medicine. It is also one of the most important constituents of rehabilitation medicine.

Nitric oxide is a recognized, well-studied and effective natural anti-inflammatory molecule that inhibits the activity of inflammation producing factors. It is capable of providing efficient effects to tame chronic inflammatory diseases.

Nitric oxide physiotherapy is a type of nonspecific treatment that applies natural or artificial physical factors upon human body. It promotes the formation of nitric oxide. Through ample level of the produced nitric oxide it then improves blood circulation, stimulates autoimmune mechanism, adjusts nervous system functions and consequently achieves the goal of disease treatment and prevention.

Three: Nitric Oxide Physiotherapy - Vibration Bed Technique

Nitric oxide vibration bed emits vibration motion and vibrates the human body with a frequency of up to140 times per minute. During the treatment of 30 to 45 minutes on vibration bed, beneficial nitric oxide is released and helps to improve circulation and increases agility of joints. It can also help to reduce pain and inflammation between muscle and bones.

The nitric oxide vibration bed of physiotherapy enhances physical fitness, prevents diseases and stimulates self-recovery mechanisms. It especially possesses a unique curing effect for limb dysfunction and recovery effect for cardiopulmonary symptoms. It is a noninvasive yet effective treatment without need of drug use. Its effectiveness is supported with positive testimonies and valid experimental results from a wide range of scientific research.

Mechanism of nitric oxide vibration bed

Nitric oxide vibration bed can vibrate the body from head to toe at a vibration frequency of up to140 times per minute. Such repeated acceleration and deceleration of movement can increase pulsing in the vascular systems. The systematic increase of pulsation in vascular endothelial regions stimulates hemoglobin activity and increases nitric oxide release in the blood flow. It subsequently improves the health and internal function of human body. For the weak and the sick, it is beneficial for their health to experience this non-invasive whole body treatment. People who need rehabilitation due to injury can also benefit from such treatment, and it reduces their needs of drug use and may prevent the need for surgery.

The experimental results showed that the vibration bed generates an additional vibration frequency at small scale that affects the endothelial cells of the whole body. It reduces the bonding ability of hemoglobin to nitric oxide, and helps to release nitric oxide into peripheral tissues, causing vasodilatation. Such mechanism helps to fight against hemoperfusion decline caused by heme elimination of

192

nitric oxide. It also helps to regulate blood flow and blood pressure. This process is called the shearing stress of the pulsation. The phenomenon increases blood flow, and helps to improve the overall circulation and function of the whole body.

Clinical effect of nitric oxide vibration bed

1. Therapeutic effect: It can be used to improve symptoms of arthritis and fibromyalgia.

2. Preventive effect: It not only helps to cure diseases, it also helps to protect the heart and slows down myocardial ischemia. It improves angina patients' exercise endurance and prevents unpredictable yet lethal myocardial infarction.

3. Effect in rehabilitation: Early application of physiotherapy can promote speedy recovery from injuries, and prevents complications. It initiates the body's repair system that has a significant effect on physical strength and independent living capability.

Four: Outlook

Nowadays, self healthcare methods originating from the source of natural medicine has become a mainstream method in the world's trend of health consciousness. Physiotherapy will also play an important role in the conventional aspects of disease prevention and sub-health status improvement. The innovative nitric oxide vibration bed not only is suitable for individuals, this modern medical instrument is also suitable for family use. The vibration bed will play a significant role in disease prevention and sub-health status improvement.

Chapter Seven
Achieving Longevity with Nitric Oxide

Everyone hopes for good health and longevity. For our ancestors, the ideal for longevity was "maximum 120 years, average 100, or at least 80". However, due to various reasons, many are unable to reach even the most basic level of longevity. The main reason for this is a lack of lifestyle habits that enable us to "complete the natural span of life".

So how can we achieve true longevity? Throughout history, man has continuously hunted for the secrets for health and longevity, and clues to the secrets of longevity have often been reached in unexpected places. Indeed, there appear to be some areas of the world where longevity can not only be achieved, but is common as well. Through decades of research, the WHO has designed an area of longevity as an area which has seven healthy elderly persons aged above 100 years for every 100,000 people in the local population. According to the statistics of WHO, there are five "regions of longevity" identifiable in the world today.: Okinawa Island in Japan, Sago Island in Greece, Campodimele in Italy, Hunza in Pakistan, and Bama of Guangxi in China.

According to the statistics of WHO, the ratio of individuals aged above 100 in these regions is 30/100000, far higher than average 7/100000! Through extensive study, scientists have identified four major secrets for health and longevity that each of these areas share: the populace of each area has healthy diets, they take part in regular exercise, they demonstrate a generally relaxed attitude towards life and live in a superior natural environment. In the "regions of longevity" in the world, none of the four secrets of health are dispensable, so how exactly do each of these secrets play a role in promoting longevity in these regions?

Healthy diet: eat more vegetables, fruit and coarse cereals

Since food is the first necessity of man, no one can do without food. As scientific statistical data indicate, in his whole life, one person must consume approximately 12,600 kilograms of grain, 4,250 kilograms of meat, 5,000 kilograms of vegetables and fruit, more than 1,000 kilograms of different snacks and more than 50 kilograms of condiments! Alongside these essential foodstuffs, it is also necessary to consume various beverages in similarly vast quantities. Studies of the diets of individuals residing in the top five villages of longevity each showed remarkable characteristics. When viewed within the framework of modern nutrition, these diets proved to be highly scientific and in line with current standards of high quality nutrition. In each area, people consumed large quantities of vegetables and fruit and relying on coarse cereals, complemented by a highly varied diet. In each of the regions, the population had maintained these dietary habits for generations.

Scientific exercise: work and exercise for life

As follow-up research on the global five major villages of longevity shows, daily scientific aerobic exercise is critical for health and longevity. People who maintain traditional lifestyles on Okinawa Island are almost all farmers or fishermen, working heavily outdoors every day. By growing crops and fishing offshore, they achieve an extremely high rate of regular exercise and are known to work in fields even at the age of 80. In addition to fishing offshore, people living on Sago Island in the Mediterranean Sea often have to walk up and down 387 stone steps several times. People living in Campodimele of Apennine Peninsula ensure an adequate amount of exercise by harvesting crops and falling trees on a regular basis. In Campodimele, it is quite normal for elderly individuals of more than 80 years to participate in hunting. For people living in Hunza in the Karakoram Range, the traditional sport of Polo remains popular. Polo has been played in the region for one thousand years and the whole body work-out that it provides is a potent weapon among the population in the fight to keep fit and healthy. Bama of Guangxi in China is surrounded by high mountains, where people have to climb mountains to grow crops. Locals also work at least 8 hours per day, thereby ensuring adequate aerobic exercise.

Calm mood: optimistic for life and full of love

In 2010, American scientists published the results of a scientific study conducted over a period of three years. Their research on 700 healthy elderly people aged above 100 explained the secrets of their longevity: an open-minded character, infrequent anxiety and anger, and a lifelong placid disposition. Chinese nationals may be reminded of the master of Traditional Chinese Medicine Lu Guangshen, who is aged 84, but looks only about 50 years old, and still has dark hair. When asked about the secrets of his youthful looks, Master Lu has said: "I am constantly carefree." Likewise, people from the global top five villages of longevity all have an optimistic outlook, are live lives enriched by love and seldom worry excessively about anything. It is clear that the path to longevity is the same whether in China or in any country in the world

People from Okinawa prefer a low-pressure, relaxed lifestyle, and have developed a close social community to ensure that they live in an atmosphere of warmth and love. People from Sago attach great importance to family life and their communities are known for their vast network of family relationships as well as being good at expressing their emotion and not suppressing their feelings. Due to a happy family environment and a low-pressure life, the inhabitants of Sago are generally of a pleasant and easy-going nature. People of Campodimele also live peacefully and are blissfully free of pressure in their daily lives. As believers of Islam, the people of Hunza see living as part of a mutually supportive society is one of the most important doctrines by which they live their lives. Their lifestyle is also carefree. People of Baba living in the hometown of folk songs in China are fond of expressing their emotions by singing in the fields. They live an easy life, spending their spare time playing mahjong and chess, practicing calligraphy and gathering together to sing songs. Through these lifestyle habits, they are able to release mental pressure, stay mentally flexible, internally satisfied and emotionally stable. This is the key of each of these groups to maintaining their health and longevity.

Superior natural environment: high content of oxygen and strong - antioxidation capacity.

Through extensive research, scientists have reached the following conclusions: a superior living environment can increase human life by 10~20 years. Greenish grass and forest, good climate, fresh air, adequate oxygen, non-polluted water sources and well-ventilated residences which allow exposure to sunlight are all factors that promote longevity. Upon investigating, it is observed that all the villages of longevity in the world are in a unique natural environment, unspoiled and with minimal pollution levels. With a high content of oxygen per m3 of air, it is honored as "bar of natural oxygen". Furthermore, in each of the regions of longevity, the environment is natural and remote, with mountains and water, good climate, fertile land, and clear and fresh spring water. Philosopher Heidegger said: man should dwell in a poetic way. Today, the idea of living an unfettered lifestyle at one with nature among green mountains and near clear water represents the ideal human living environment for many people.

"NO regimen" helps people throughout the world to "complete the natural span of life"

It has always been a project for scientists to understand how the lifestyles of the inhabitants of the "regions of longevity" might be popularized elsewhere. Yet due to economic development and centralization of populations in numerous countries, it is practically impossible for everyone to live in an environment that achieves the conditions of live in the regions of longevity, meaning that the insights into achieving longevity that these regions provide have their limits for the practical considerations of the vast majority of people in the world. According to several scientific studies, since the four major secrets of longevity are all associated directly with nitric oxide, people who maintain in vivo nitric oxide at a reasonable concentration are in fact unknowingly accessing the four secrets of longevity. According to the research on the global top five villages of longevity, a so-called

198

"nitric oxide regimen" can be observed, of which the foundations are "rational diet, scientific exercises, targeted nutritional supplements and emotional composure".

1) Rational diet

The healthier diet, the more nitric oxide human produces. So what constitutes a healthy diet?

Firstly, it is important to eat a good variety of vegetables and fruits, for they provide significant quantities of antioxidants. Through various biological mechanisms, these antioxidants protect human cells against oxidation and prevent in vivo nitric oxide from being damaged.

Secondly, avoid eating foods that contain saturated fatty acids, trans-fatty acids and cholesterol such as fatty meat, red meat, deserts, cheese and potato chips, reduce the in vivo generation of free radicals and control, at the source place, the amount of free radicals attacking nitric oxide.

In my (Murad) daily meals, I will take in a lot of vegetables and fruit, bean products, yoghurt, fish, hard nuts and other food rich in arginine, but never anything sweet.

2) Scientific motion

Through research, scientists discovered that consecutive or repeated aerobic exercise can produce nitric oxide in two ways: (1) aerobic exercise can regulate NOS at the vascular endothelium; the more NOS is present at vascular endothelium, the more nitric oxide will be produced. (2) Through regular aerobic exercise, blood circulation increases, directly causing the vascular endothelium to produce more nitric oxide.

3) Targeted nutritional supplements

Since our way of living has changed to a great extent, it is impossible to meet the environmental standard for villages: we all experience high work pressure, little time for exercising, copious available junk food and frequent exposure to air pollution, all of which will damage in vivo nitric oxide and limit our capacity to avoid cardio-cerebrovascular diseases. If you live in this way, it is better to take nutritional supplements to increase the concentration of your in vivo nitric oxide, mainly through amino acids and antioxidants that can be obtained from health-care products. Amino acid supplements are composed of L-citrulline and L-arginine. Vitamin C, Vitamin E, folic acid and other antioxidants can also promote the generation of nitric oxide.

4) Emotional composure

Achieving a calm emotional state will have the effect of relaxing the muscles. Blood circulation will speed up, while faster blood flow velocity will stimulate vascular endothelial cells to produce more nitric oxide. Therefore, by maintaining emotional composure, one can help his/her body to produce more nitric oxide.

These are the scientific reasons behind the secrets of these villages. The "nitric oxide regimen" is based on these scientific principles and is suitable for people throughout the world. For those who do not live in a superior natural environment like those of the five regions of longevity, but wish to extend their life span significantly, the "nitric oxide regimen" can help them to "complete the natural span of life"!

PART FIVE
GROUPS IN NEED OF NITRIC OXIDE

As a kind of nutritional supplement, nitric oxide is involved in the circulation and metabolism of different systems in the human body and shows an extremely important effect for health. What kind of people need to supplement nitric oxide? As studies show, those in need to supplement include: elderly, mental workers, post-menopausal women, smokers as a group, alcohol drinkers as a group, obese subjects as a group, and hypothyroid persons. Obviously, there are large groups.

Chapter One
Elderly

Different cultures define age in different ways. Since human life is a process of gradual change, the boundaries between the young and the old are often rather ambiguous. According to some people, being a grandfather or grandmother denotes old age; according to others, retirement symbolizes an elderly age. The WHO defines the elderly as those aged more than 60, while in some western developed countries, that age is 65. In ancient China, the age of 50 was once used to mark old age. Biologically speaking, old age may be characterized by a slowing metabolism, lower immunity, and deteriorating physiological functions that increase the probability of illness.

Common elderly diseases

The elderly suffer more diseases than the young and these diseases have their own unique features. This is mainly because human tissue structure and various physiological functions begin to deteriorate, thus leading to a decline in physical capability among elderly people.

Generally speaking, diseases that affect the elderly display the following three characteristics:

1) Specific diseases for the elderly

Most diseases that are specific to the elderly such as senile dementia, senile psychosis, presbyopia, cerebral atherosclerosis and cerebral stroke are due to hypofunction and dysfunction. The risk of contracting any of these diseases grows with old age.

2) Common diseases for the elderly

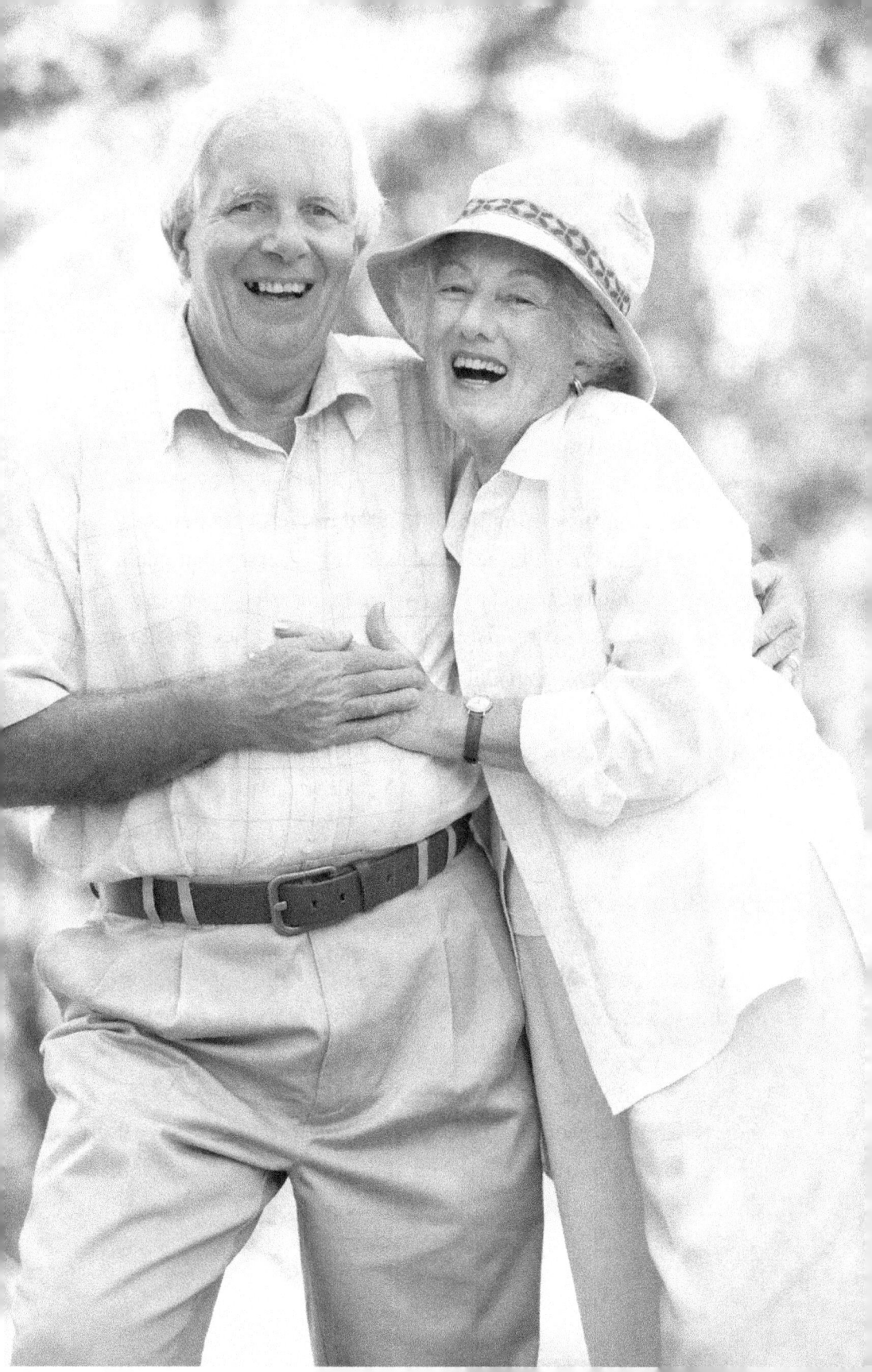

Such diseases may take place during middle age and during presenile old age as well as during senile old age. However, diseases become more common or worse in their effects during the senile period. They are closely linked with pathological aging, declining physical immunity, long-term stress or declining physique due to diseases suffered when young or middle aged, and include conditions such as hypertension, coronary heart disease, diabetes, malignant tumors, gout, paralysis, osteoarthritis, chronic bronchitis, emphysema, long-derived cardiopathy, cataracts, elderly osteoporosis, pneumonia, hyperlipidemia, cervical spondylosis, prostatic hypertrophy, etc.

3) Diseases among young, middle-aged and elderly people

Due to hypofunction during old age, many diseases that occur at any age display unique characteristics when manifested among the elderly. For example, people of different ages may contract pneumonia, but the elderly frequently display non-typical symptoms and suffer from even worse conditions. Pneumonia is a common cause of death in the elderly. To take another example, young, middle-aged and elderly people may all suffer from digestive ulcers, but it is easier for the elderly to develop complications or cancers.

Prevention and control of disease in old age

Prevention and control of diseases is one of the important measures for health-care of the elderly. Since cellular and organic tissues deteriorate with age, their ability to adapt declines, resistance decreases and incidence of disease increases. The diseases to which elderly Chinese people are most vulnerable are tumors, hypertension and coronary heart disease, chronic bronchitis and pneumonia, cholelithiasis (gallstones), prostatic hypertrophy, femoral fractures and diabetes, etc., while the most common causes of death among the elderly are pneumonia, cerebral hemorrhage, lung cancer, gastric cancer, acute myocardial infarction, etc.

To avoid these conditions, the elderly may pay attention to the following guidelines for diet in old age:

1) Complete food

Maintain a varied diet including coarse cereals, meat, poultry, egg and milk, land and water vegetables, dry and fresh fruit, fish, shellfish, shrimp and crab, mushrooms and seafood. Elderly individuals suffering hypertension, coronary heart disease may still eat lean meat and milk without any adverse effects and should eat more beans as well.

2) Light diet

As the elderly have reduced sense of taste, they are often especially fond of oily and fried foods. However, such foods cannot be easily digested, and should be consumed in moderation. According to TCM, excessive consumption of fat and sweet foods will easily cause excess moisture and sputum to be produced, and may even release toxins. Therefore, it is better to stick to a light, low fat diet. With cereals as nutrition, fruit and vegetables as supplement and meat as assistance, it is possible to ensure the supply of different nutrients as well as keep excrement unobstructed. Often calorie intake in the elderly is decreased.

3) Temperate diet

Due to the poor adaptability of the gastrointestinal tract, the elderly should avoid diets that will cause digestive disorders, air and blood stasis and food corruption, as these will lead to symptoms such as abdominal distension, diarrhea and eructation and can even result in death due to acute gastritis or inducing myocardial infarction for death.

4) Food should be soft and tender

With worn, loose and lost teeth, the ability to chew food effectively decreases with age, while a drop in the secretion of various digestive enzymes over time means that digestive capacity also deteriorates. Therefore, it is necessary to cut food into small pieces and cook it thoroughly. Meat can be prepared into meat emulsion, the young leaves of vegetables can be used. Cooking should be mostly prepared by braising, stewing, steaming and boiling for a short time. Try to avoid any fried food and stimulating condiments. Additionally, attention should also be given to presentation, flavor and taste to increase appetite and promote digestion.

5) Frequent meals in less quantity

After reaching old age, the capacity of the liver to synthesize glycogen is weak, leading to lower glycogen reserves and feelings of hunger and dizziness. Therefore, before sleeping, after getting up or between two meals, it is appropriate for the elderly to eat a moderate amount of food as refreshment. Generally, five regular smaller meals are suitable, and the amount served for each meal should be carefully controlled. No snacks, especially sweet food, should be taken between meals, in order to avoid affecting the appetite and causing digestive dysfunction.

6) Appropriate temperature

Due to decreasing saliva secretion and deteriorating resistance function of oral mucosa, the elderly should not consume excessively hot food, as this may be one of the main causes for esophagus cancer. On the other hand, excessive cold food can easily injure gastric health. In TCM, the adage that "raw and cold food impairs spleen and hard substances are difficult to digest" is highly applicable in this situation.

7) Fresh food

It is better to avoid rotten fish, meat or fruit, acescent oil, moldy peanuts, cereals or beans and food kept overnight to avoid food poisoning or even cancer.

8) More fruit and vegetables

The elderly should make sure they eat more fresh fruit and vegetables to ensure the adequate supply of vitamins and minerals. Pectin and cellulose are effective in promoting gastrointestinal peristalsis and can prevent the retention of feces in the intestine, and also help lower the risk of constipation, diverticulitis and intestinal tumors. Additionally, eating kelp, laver and other marine plant food, will contribute to the prevention of atherosclerosis and cerebrovascular diseases.

9) Adequate water content

Soup, both thick and of normal consistency, and mashed vegetables for the elderly will supplement water as well as benefit digestion.

Nitric oxide and the control of disease in the elderly

The elderly should ensure that they supplement their diets with nitric oxide in order to guard against the various old-age specific cardio-cerebrovascular diseases, immune system diseases, and nervous system diseases.

1) Nitric oxide protects vessels

Nitric oxide is helpful in removing the refuse adhered to vascular inter walls and quickly repair vascular endothelium so that free radicals cannot attack the vascular endothelium when it is injured, thus protecting vessels and restoring vessel elasticity.

2) Nitric oxide reduces hypertension

Nitric oxide can dilate vascular smooth muscle and lower blood pressure.

3) Nitric oxide lowers hyperlipemia

Nitric oxide can effectively inhibit the sythesis of LDL, thereby reducing LDL levels in the blood within a short time and allowing cholesterol and TG in blood to decrease accordingly. Additionally, nitric oxide can promote the synthesis of HDL so that cholesterol and TG in blood are promptly released to complete the function of lowering fat levels.

4) Nitric oxide improves diabetic angiopathy

As many studies have shown, by adding L- arginine in the diet of diabetic animals, it is possible to increase the synthesis of in vivo nitric oxide in diabetic animals thereby delaying the incidence of diabetic angiopathy or improving the condition of patients with diabetic angiopathy. According to recent research, exercise can cause nitric oxide synthesis in the body of diabetic patients to increase and therefore delay injury to vascular endothelium. These results have provided a basis for the clinical work to prevent and control the injury to diabetic vascular endothelium by increasing in patients the in vivo nitric oxide.

5) Nitric oxide alleviates cerebral thrombus

The formation period and ultra-early period of acute cerebral thrombus, is closely linked with the decrease of nitric oxide content; upon formation of thrombus and during brain edema, nitric oxide may be involved in injuring brain tissues. Nitric oxide also increases blood clots from forming.

Nitric oxide also functions to improve conditions in patients suffering from stroke, hemiplegia, senile dementia, memory deterioration, sexual dysfunction, insomnia, melancholy and specific cancers.

The immune system strengthening function of nitric oxide means that it is an effective weapon for combating bacteria, viruses, tumor cells and other pathogens.

For the nervous system, nitric oxide acts a transmitter of neural signals and can enhance cerebral blood flow. It may also be associated with the development of cerebral cells, learning and memory process of cerebral cells, secretion of pituitary hormones such as vasopressin and oxytocin, protection of cerebral cells against toxins and regulation of cerebral blood supply in cerebral ischemia.

Chapter Two
Mental Workers as a Group

The brain has a complicated structure, a heavy workload and a highly active metabolism. It therefore requires a considerable range of nutritional substances to ensure its continuous normal function. For any mental activity, cerebral cells require a huge amount of oxygen. The human brain weighs only 1.4kg, but its oxygen consumption shares 1/5~1/4 of systemic oxygen consumption. Being a big

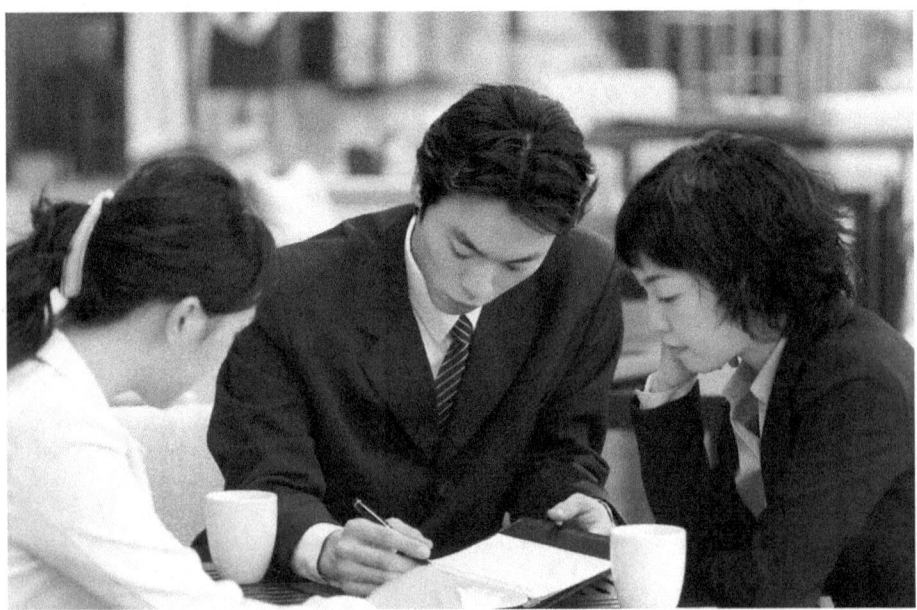

"account" for most oxygen requirement in the body, its energy needs to be supplied all from carbohydrate, as the brain cannot store energy by itself.

In case of intensive mental activity, the necessary glucose and oxygen consumption will increase accordingly. Therefore, those working in cognitively intensive fields require a higher quality of diet than those working in physical vocations. To function normally, cerebral cells require a large quantity of oxygen and carbohydrate. The major components of the brain are protein, fat (mainly lecithin), as well as Vitamin B1 and nicotinic acid which have the greatest effect on the brain. Therefore, to meet the energy requirements of the brain, a

sufficient supply of protein and vitamins is required. Nitric oxide can help the human body to maintain a smooth flow of blood and transmit arterial blood rich in oxygen and energy to the brain so as to relieve mental fatigue. For this reason, workers in cognitively intensive fields benefit greatly from nitric oxide supplements.

Chapter Three
Menopausal Women

The menopause is a transitional stage for women between their fertile period and old age, and consequently entails significant physiological change. No matter when it starts and how long it lasts, the menopause can be divided into three stages , namely the premenopause , menopause and postmenopause, according to the functional decline of the ovaries. During the menopause, more than 90% of women will experience symptoms that affect personal health and life quality to varying extents. Therefore, during the menopause, every woman should pay attention to their health to ensure that this period of transition in their lives is completed as smoothly as possible.

Symptoms of the menopause

1) Around age 30: significant abnormal phenomena as mottling, darkness, large and rough sweat pores, and chronic acne can be observed in the skin.

2) 30~40 years: endocrine disorders, such as dry vulva, declining sexual desire, significant aging and weakening of the female secondary sexual organ and other symptoms may occur.

3) 40~55 years: menopausal symptoms as insomnia, dreaminess, night sweats, hectic fever, irritability and testiness, declining energy and physical strength, memory deterioration, and osteoporosis can be observed.

4) Over 55 years: renal function declines sharply and the ovarian function is decreased.

Four major symptoms of female menopause:

1) Fevers (hot flushes) are a symptom encountered frequently by females during the menopause.

2) Cardiac palpitations are one of the most common symptoms during menopause.

3) Exhibition of abnormal mental and neural symptoms.

4) Soreness and back pain are the early symptoms of osteoporosis for menopausal women.

Menopausal women are observed to experience inadequate secretion of estrogen and poor formation of bone tradecula. During this period, lack of Vitamin D may lead to poor absorption of calcium and the combination of the two will result in osteoporosis. Through the secretion of ovarian granular cells, nitric oxide can regulate estrogen levels in the body so as to improve female menopausal symptoms.

Chapter Four
Smokers as a Group

Harmful substances in cigarettes: it is a well-known fact that smoking harms health. Cigarettes release mainly tars and carbon monoxide when lit, in addition to numerous harmful substances that can be basically classified into six major categories:

1) Aldehydes, nitrite and alkenes, all of which stimulate the respiratory tract.

2) Nicotine, which can stimulate the sympathetic nerves and cause damage to vascular intima.

3) Amine, cyanide and heavy metals, all of which are toxic.

4) BaP, arsenic, cadmium, monomethylhydrazine, aminophenol, and other substances, which are all carcinogenic.

5) Phenolic compounds and formalin, which can accelerate the onset of cancer.

6) CO, which can reduce the capacity of erythrocytes to transmit oxygen to the whole body.

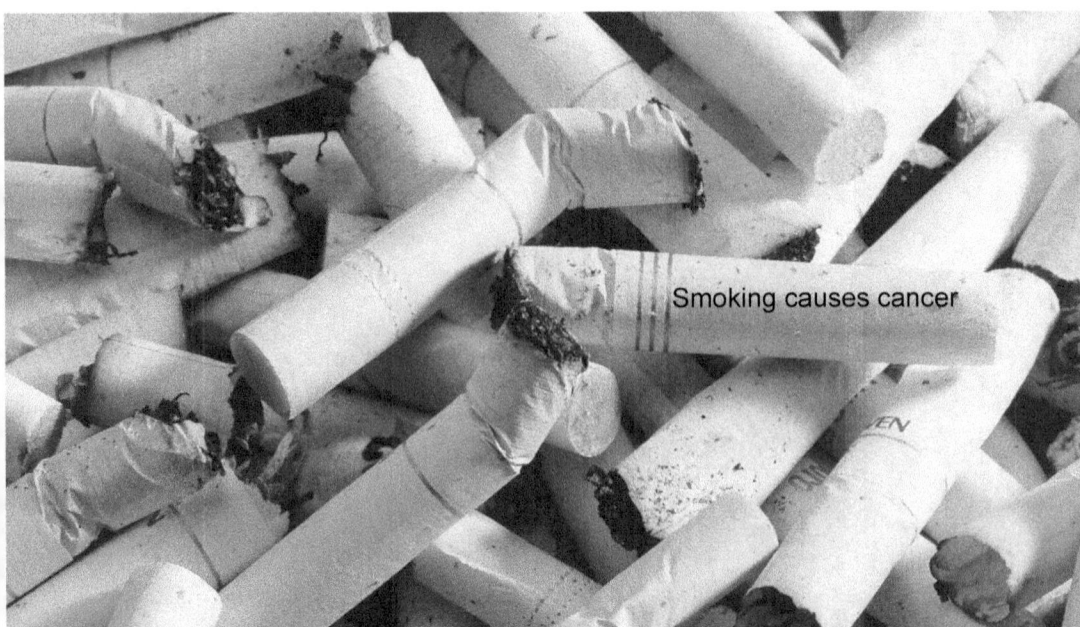

Smoking causes cancer

It is universally recognized that smoking causes cancer. According to the epidemiological survey, smoking is one of the main causes of lung cancer, especially squamous epithelial carcinoma and small cell undifferentiated carcinoma. Among those who smoke, the risk of contracting lung cancer is 1.3 times that of non-smokers. If one smokes more than 35 cigarettes per day, the risk is 45 times higher than that for non-smokers. The mortality rate of lung cancer for smokers is 10~13 times higher than that of non-smokers. 85% lung cancer related deaths are due to smoking. If exposed to chemical carcinogenic substances (such as asbestos, nickel, uranium and arsenic), smokers will have an even higher risk of lung cancer. The polycyclic aromatic hydrocarbons in tobacco and smoke can produce cellular toxins and induce a mutating effect on the genes. In the body of smokers, the concentration of hydroxylase is higher than that of non-smokers. Smoking can reduce the activity of natural immune cells, thus weakening the body's ability to deal with tumor cells. For this reason, smoking leads to the higher incidence of various cancers of the lung, pancreas and bladder and other tissues. The incidence of laryngeal cancer for smokers is more than one dozen times higher than that for non-smokers. The incidence of bladder cancer increases by 3 times, which may be explained by the presence β-naphthamine in cigarette smoke. Moreover, smoking is also associated with the onset of lip cancer, tongue cancer, oral cancer, esophagus cancer, gastric cancer, colon cancer, pancreatic cancer, renal cancer and cervical cancer. According to clinical research and animal experiments, carcinogenic substances in cigarette smoke can also affect fetus development through the placenta, leading to a higher risk of cancer in the children of those who smoke during pregnancy.

Effects on cardio-cerebrovascular health

According to many studies, smoking leads to a higher risk of many diseases such as coronary heart disease, hypertension, and cerebrovascular diseases. As statistical data indicates, among patients of coronary heart disease and hypertension, 75% have a history of smoking. The mortality rate of coronary heart disease in smokers is 6 times higher than in non-smokers. And incidence of myocardial infarction is 2-6 times higher. It has also been observed that coronary artery atherosclerosis lesions are more common and more severe among smokers than among non-smokers. For smokers suffering from hypertension and high cholesterol, the incidence of coronary heart disease increases by 9~12 times. Furthermore, 30%~40% of cardiovascular disease related deaths are caused by smoking, with a positive correlation between mortality rate and number of cigarettes smoked on a regular basis. Nicotine and CO in cigarette smoke are major health hazards universally recognized primary causes of coronary artery atherosclerosis. However its actual mechanism is not yet clear. According to most specialists, change of blood lipid and abnormality of platelet function and blood flow may play an important role. HDL cholesterol can stimulate the generation of prostacyclin in vascular endothelial cells that are effective substances for dilating vessels and inhibiting platelets from aggregation. Smoking can damage vascular endothelial cells, and can result in decreasing levels of serum HDL cholesterol, increase of cholesterol, and declining levels of prostacyclin in vascular endothelial cells, thus leading to the contraction of the peripheral vascular and coronary artery, thickening of the vascular walls, luminal stenosis and blood flow slowdown, leading to hypoxia of myocardium. Nicotine can also

216

promote the aggregation of platelets. CO in cigarette smoke combines with hemoglobin to form carboxyhemoglobin, which affects the oxygen carrying function of erythrocytes, resulting in tissue hypoxia which causes coronary artery spasms. Hypoxia of tissues leads to the increase of compensatory erythrocytes and results in increasing blood viscosity. Apart from the above, smoking can cause an increase in plasma fibrous proteins, resulting in coagulation system dysfunction. Smoking can also affect the metabolism of arachidonic acid, leading to a decrease in the rate of prostacyclinin generation in vascular endothelial cells and a relative increase of thrombus A2. This leads to increasing vasoconstriction and platelet aggregation. All the above may promote the incidence and development of coronary heart disease. Due to myocardium hypoxia, myocardium stress is potentiated and the ventricle fibrillation threshold declines. Therefore, smokers having coronary heart disease easily suffer from arrhythmia and have a higher risk of sudden death.

It is reported that the risk of stroke for smokers is 2~3.5 times higher than that for non-smokers. For smokers suffering from hypertension, the risk of suffering a stroke will increase by nearly 20 times. Additionally, it is easy for smokers to suffer from atheriosclerosis obliterans and occlusive thromboendarteritis. Smoking can lead to chronic obstructive pulmonary disease (COPD) and eventually to pulmonary heart disease.

Effects on the respiratory tract

Smoking is one of the causes for chronic bronchitis, emphysema and chronic airway obstruction. According to the discovery of experimental studies, long-term smoking can cause the cilia of bronchial mucosa to shorten and become damaged, which affects the removing function of cilia. Additionally, with hyperplasia and hypertrophy of submucosal gland and increased secretion of mucus as well as change in components, it is easy for the bronchiole to become congested. In several experiments, it has been shown that extensive contact with smoke and dust can lead to emphysema changes. According to the findings of one research project by CMU Respiratory Disease Institute, smokers' lower respiratory tract phagocyte (AM), neutrophilic granulocyte (PMN) and elasticity protease show a significant increase as compared to non-smokers. This mechanism may be attributable to the stimulation of smoke particles and harmful gases, which activated the lower respiratory tract phagocyte system, The activated phagocyte can then release elastic protease as well as release neutrophil chemokines, shifting neutrophil from capillaries to the lungs. Activated phagocytes also releases phagocyte growth factor, attracting fibroblasts, while neutrophils releases a massive amount of toxic free radicals and proteolytic enzymes including elastase and collagenase, elastin, mucopolysaccharide protein, basement membrane and collagen fiber which can lead to damage and interstitial fibrosis in the alveolae. It is reported that in USA, there were 13 million cases of COPD in 1986 and over 90,000 persons died in 1991 mainly due to smoking. Incidence of winter cough for smokers is 2~4 times higher than that for non-smokers, and it is proportional to the amount of cigarettes smoked over the years, while patients often show such symptoms as chronic coughing, expectoration and difficult respiration in exercising. As tests on pulmonary functions show, the respiratory tract is blocked, while lung compliance, pulmonary ventilation function and diffusing function decline leading to a decrease in oxygen content in arterial blood. Even young smokers without any symptoms may also experience some pulmonary dysfunction. COPD easily leads to spontaneous pneumothorax, and smokers often suffer from chronic pharyngitis and bronchitis.

Effects on the digestive tract

Smoking may cause an increase in the secretion of gastric acid, generally by 91.5% more than non-smokers, and can inhibit the secretion of sodium bicarbonate in the pancreas, resulting in ulcers caused by excessive exposure to acid in the duodenum. Tobacco nicotine can decrease the tension of the pyloric sphincter and causes easy reflux of bile, thus weakening the defending factors of gastric and duodenal mucosa, promoting the incidence of chronic inflammation and ulcer, and delaying recovery from existing ulcers. Additionally, smoking can reduce the tension of the lower esophageal sphincter, which leads to reflux esophagitis.

Others

Smoking is even more harmful to females than to males. Women who smoke may experience menstrual disorders, conception difficulties, ectopic pregnancies, low estrogen levels, osteoporosis and early menopause. For pregnant women, smoking may easily lead to miscarriages, fetus development problems and low birth weight in newborn babies. Other complications such as premature delivery, stillbirth, premature separation of placenta and placenta previa are all linked to smoking. Smoking during pregnancy may increase the risk of fetus mortality prior to and after birth as well as the incidence of congenital cardiomyopathy. The hazards mentioned above are due to the presence of harmful substances in cigarette smoke as CO, which enter the blood of the fetus and form carboxyhemoglobin, resulting in hypoxia. Nicotine also causes vascoconstriction, reducing the supply of blood and nutrition to the fetus, consequently affecting the normal growth and development of the fetus. For women, 90% of lung cancer cases, 75% of COPD cases and 25% of coronary heart disease cases are linked to smoking. The probability for smoking women to die of breast cancer is 25% higher than non-smoking women. As studies prove, nicotine has the effect of reducing sex hormone secretion and lowering sperm count and decreasing the quality of sperm, thus lowering chances of conception. Smoking may also inhibit the functions of the testes, cause a decline of male sexual function and even male infertility. For the elderly, smoking causes macular degeneration, possibly because atherosclerosis and platelet aggregation increases, promoting partial hypoxia. According to recent research in the USA, smoking in an environment with high noise levels will cause permanent hearing decline and even deafness.

Thanks to its reputation as a safe and reliable treatment, nitric oxide therapy is highly praised by smokers throughout the world:

Nitric oxide helps smokers to avoid cancer. Using nitric oxide, leukocytes are not only able to kill a series of pathogens such as bacteria, fungi and mycoplasma, but are also effective at resisting tumors. As nitric oxide can induce the dying and decaying course of cells, scientists are now conducting experiments to see if nitric oxide can be used to inhibit the growth of tumors.

Nitric oxide helps smokers to prevent sexual dysfunction. By dilating vessels in erection tissues, nitric oxide helps maintain penile erection. Such knowledge has been used to develop new drugs to treat impotence.

Nitric oxide helps smokers to improve respiratory disease symptoms. By analyzing the content of nitric oxide in the lungs and small intestine, it is possible to identify inflammatory diseases meaning that nitric oxide can be used for diagnosing asthma, colitis and other related diseases.

Chapter Five
Alcohol Drinkers as a Group

In daily life, people regularly consume alcoholic drinks such as beer, wine and spirits. Different alcoholic drinks have different sources, brewing processes and degrees of alcohol content. Alcoholic degree usually refers to the percentage of alcoholic content in alcoholic drinks by volume. For instance, Beijing Beer contains 5.4% alcohol; wine contains about 11%~16% alcohol, generally known as 11~16°, while spirits contain 38%—60% alcohol, while those containing 38% of alcohol are called low-alcohol spirits.

Article 7 of the China Dietary Guide advises "drinking in moderation" and in one section describes the harmful effects of excessive drinking. A limited amount of low-alcohol liquor will not be harmful, but excessive drinking and even intemperance inevitably produces some harmful effects. What kind of alcoholic drinks can therefore be consumed? And how can we limit the amount that we drink?

As extensive studies have shown, if the daily volume of alcoholic consumed is less than 24g alcohol, equal to 540ml of beer, 200ml of wine, 60ml 40°liquor, the hazard will be minimal.

Long-term drinking may lead to a shortage of various nutrients in the body. Alcoholic drinks can be metabolized and produce energy in vivo, but contain no nutrients. Firstly, excessive drinking reduces the intake of other foods containing various important nutrients (such as protein, Vitamin, minerals). Secondly, it has the effect of reducing appetite and food consumption; furthermore, long-term excessive drinking damages the intestinal mucosa and affects the absorption of nutrients by the intestines.

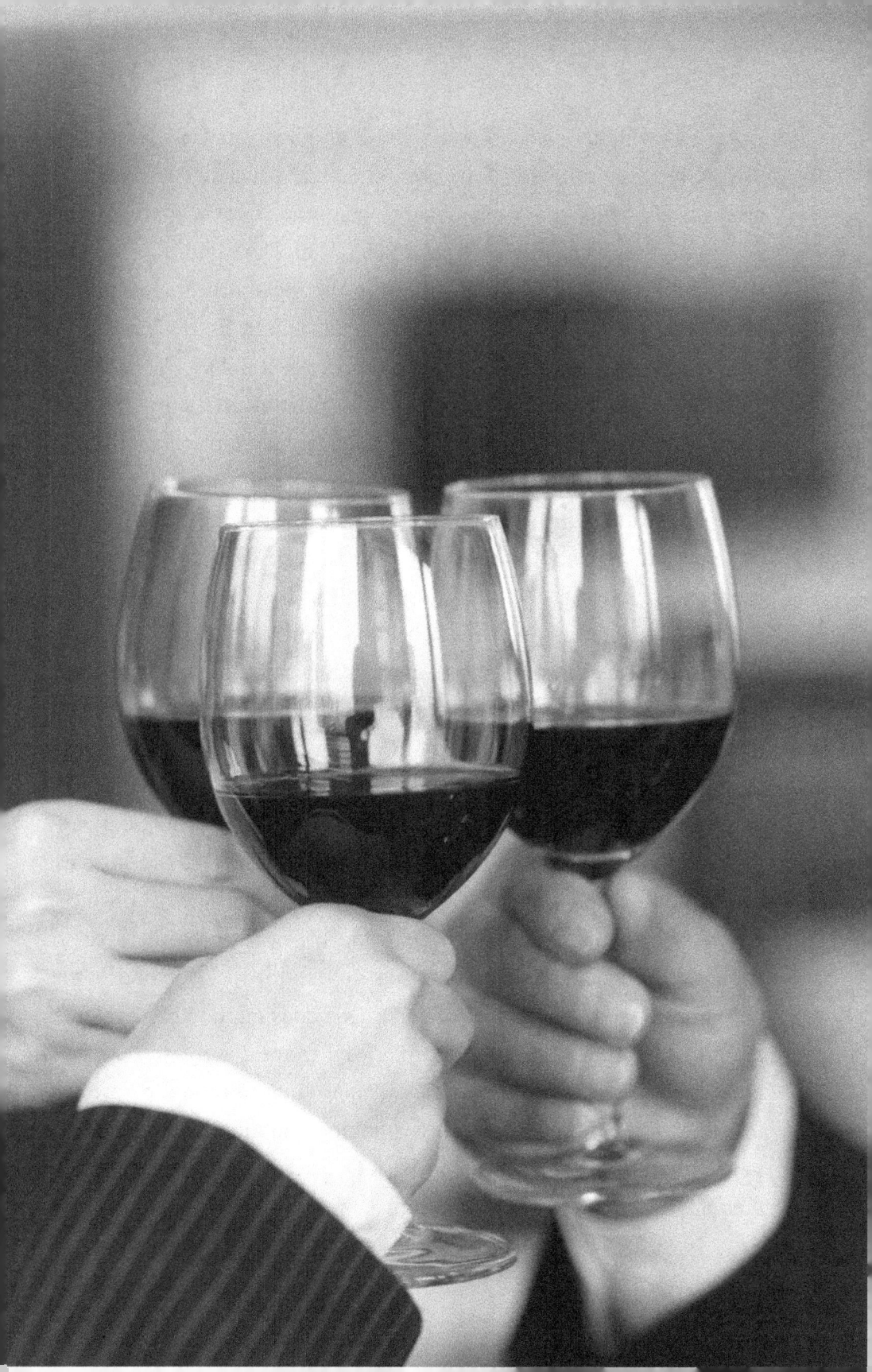

Experts have noted that excessive drinking mostly causes harm to the liver. One expert stated: "The core chemical substance of alcoholic drinks is ethyl alcohol or ethanol. The common effect of getting drunk is actually intoxication. More than 90% of alcohol entering the body is metabolized through the liver, while the metabolites and disorder of hepatocytes arising thereof are the main reason for alcoholic liver injury. Research shows that if an average of 40—80g of alcohol is consumed each day, a normal person will suffer alcoholic liver disease in 10 years; if 160g is consumed per day, hepatic cirrhosis will incur in 8~10 years. It is really a surprising figure!"

Excessive drinking affects fat metabolism. By slowing the oxidation of fatty acids, alcohol can increase the storage of dietary lipids and increase of liver fat synthesis, causing the increase of triglyceride content in serum and raise the risk of hypertriglyceidemia. Additionally, as the research of population epidemiology indicates, long-term excessive drinking will increase the risk of hypertension, cerebral stroke and may also lead to violent behavior, which may lead to other indirect forms of harm to the human body.

In recent times, the beneficial effects of wine have been frequently discussed. According to the discovery of one French report, the incidence of coronary heart disease in areas where wine is consumed in greater quantities is lower than that of other areas. However, the risk reduction of cardiomyopathy cannot be ascribed to the consumption red wine alone for certain, as consumption of vegetables and fruit is also high in the areas of France where red wine is consumed in significant quantities. It may therefore be the case that the lifestyle of wine drinkers (less smoking and more consumption of vegetables and fruits) reduces the risk of cardiovascular disease more than the properties of red wine itself.

In general, alcohol drinking has both beneficial and harmful effects towards human health. Moderate amounts of low-alcohol drinks can be beneficial for the human body, but long-term excessive drinking is harmful, especially for teenagers and pregnant women. Being in a stage of growing and development teenagers are more sensitive to hazards of alcohol, so it is advisable for teenagers not to drink alcohol excessively. The hazard of alcohol for pregnant women extends to the development of the fetus and may even cause congenital malformation, so women are strongly advised to avoid drinking during pregnancy.

As studies show, as compared to non-excessive drinkers, the incidence of oral and throat cancer among excessive drinkers increases by up to more than two times, The incidence of thyroid carcinoma increases by 30%~150%, the incidence of skin cancer by 20%~70%, and the incidence of breast cancer among women by 20%—60%. Among patients with esophageal cancer, excessive drinkers account for 60% of the total number, while non-drinkers account for only 2%. Furthermore, among patients with B-type hepatitis for whom the risk of liver cancer is already relatively high, drinking or excessive drinking, increases this risk even further.

Additionally, excessive drinking will have a damaging effect on other parts of the human body:

Excessive consumption of alcohol can cause severe damage to memory, attention span, cognitive abilities, function and emotional response. Excessive drinking will result in slurred speech, blurred vision, and a loss of balance.

Genital organs: alcohol can lower sperm count in males. As for pregnant women, even a small amount of alcohol will increase the risk of physical defects in unborn infants.

Heart: binge drinkers frequently experience injury of cardiac muscles, while fibrous tissue hyperplasia will severely impact the function of the heart.

Stomach: binge drinking can cause the stomach to exhibit symptoms of gastritis; consecutive massive intake of alcohol will lead to more severe chronic gastritis.

Some Asian people lack the gene to metabolize the oxidized aldehyde that comes from alcohol which can cause flushing of the face due to histamine release and excess nitric oxide produced in the skin.

Nitric oxide is useful for drinkers as a group:

Nitric oxide can help the liver to recover from alcohol-related damage. By regulating the blood flow of the liver, nitric oxide affects the oxidation of hepatic tissues; when nitric oxide synthesis is inhibited, blood flow of hepatic sinusoidal vessels decreases, platelets aggregate, micro thrombi are formed, leukocytes adhere, and oxidative injury to hepatic tissues can be aggravated. When nitric oxide synthesis increases, it can improve tissue ischemia and reduce oxidative injury. Nitric oxide can regulate the vascular system and blood circulation system in the body. When the endothelium sends relaxing signals to muscles in order to promote blood circulation, it will produce some nitric oxide molecules, which are very small and can easily pass through cell membranes. Perivascular smooth muscle cells will dilate upon receipt of the signal so that vessels are dilated to regulate the vascular system and blood circulation system, transmitting the oxygen-rich blood to tissues and organs.

Chapter Six
Benefits for the Beauty Conscious

For beauty-conscious women, the prospect of wrinkles, mottling and other signs of aging are the stuff of nightmares. As the body ages and is constantly exposed to the effects of the sun and external environment, the skin accumulates free radicals, which damage collagen protein in normal cellular membrane tissues and active substances, oxidizing cells, leading to formation of small fine cracks and wrinkles on the surface. The order in which areas of the body begin to wrinkle is generally as follows: forehead, upper and lower eyelid, outer canthus, the jaw area, cheek, neck, chin and mouth area. Facial wrinkles include two types: atrophic wrinkles and hypertrophic wrinkles. Atrophic wrinkling refers to any wrinkles that appear on thin, easily breakable and dry skin, such as the numerous fine wrinkles that appear around the eyes. Hypertrophic wrinkling refers to any wrinkles appearing on oily skin in a limited number and with close and deep texture, such as the wrinkles on the forehead, around lips, and on the jaw.

Latest discovery for formation of wrinkles: wrinkles, fishtail lines, fine cracks and eye tail lines are all due to uneven and subsiding collagen below the skin surface. The structure of skin can be divided into three layers: the epidermis, dermis, and subcutaneous fat. The epidermis includes collagen protein, elastin and other fibers, which provide a frame that supports the skin and helps keep it smooth and young. This layer is highly vulnerable to injury from sunlight with its UVA, UVB and ozone or other oxidants. UVA (380—420nm) can go as deep as to dermal and subcutaneous tissues, while UVB can reach only the epidermis, while ozone can generally penetrate the stratum corneum (the outermost layer of the epidermis).

Facial wrinkles can be classified into three categories: postural wrinkles, dynamic wrinkles and gravity wrinkles. 1) Postural wrinkles mostly occur as a result of the long-term extension of platysma, and are mainly found on the neck. Postural wrinkles are not necessarily all due to skin aging, but as the age increases, creases become deeper and deeper, resulting in clear wrinkles in the skin. 2) Dynamic wrinkles result from the long-term contraction of expression muscle, frontal muscle responsible for moving eyebrows, glabella lines, fishtail lines along orbicularis oculi muscle, angulus oris lines and vertical lines on orbicularis oris muscle and vertical lines of lips, major zygomatic muscle, quadratus labii superiors, buccal part and twill. 3) Gravity wrinkles are gradually created mainly due to aging of the skin, the deterioration of hypodermis fat, muscle and skeleton, together with the long-term effect of the earth's gravity. However, these wrinkles can also be classified as physiological wrinkles, pathological wrinkles, sunlight related wrinkles and aging wrinkles. Collagen protein is the elastic network structure in the skin, the loss of which will also result in wrinkles.

Collagen protein is a form of high-molecular protein, present in the skin, skeleton, teeth and tendons. Its main physiological function is as an adhesive substance for connective tissues. In terms of skin, jointly with elastic fiber, it acts as a stable and powerful support structure for the dermal layer.

If the human body were compared to the concrete framework of a building, the function of collagen would be broadly analogous to that of an adhesive agent. It is essential for maintaining the elasticity of skin and muscles. As the body ages, female collagen protein will be gradually be lost. As this happens, dermal tissues will collapse, resulting in wrinkles, skin will become loose and droop, skin will become oily, and sweat pores whose elasticity cannot be restored will become large rough and big; free radicals and dark pigment will build in skin cavities.

For females, supplementing collagen protein not only can remove wrinkles, but can also keep the skin white and moist, while removing black thimbles and eye haustra, eliminating plaques and enlarging the breasts. Collagen protein can restructure and repair dermal collagen proteins and support skin cells.

As the latest research proves, different cells in skin are observed with nitric oxide pathways, including keratinocyte, melanocyte, langerhans cell, fibroblast and endothelial cells. Nitric oxide is effective in such cells, and is associated with processes that deal with skin inflammation, immune skin disease and skin cancer. Sweat on the skin surface contains significant quantities of nitrate, which can generate NO upon acidification and reduction, and is not inhibited by NOS inhibitors. Such chemical synthesis provides the skin with a protective mechanism to regulate the growth of bacteria and prevent pathogenic infection. By promoting the synthesis of fibroblasts, nitric oxide can reduce pathological and physiological sequela in the early

stages of inflammation and late stages of hyperplasis and during the tissue forming stage. Research has also shown that the NO synthesis of fibroblasts in hypertrophic scar tissues decreases. Nitric oxide can also affect the functions of langerhans cells, such as microbe extermination and the presentation of antigens to combat cellular viruses; it can also affect adjacent keratinocytes and melanocytes (since langerhans cell (LC) is quite close to black cells in the dermis, nitric oxide produced from LC also affects these cells).

Nitric oxide and skin

The human skin is the outer covering of the body. In humans, it is the largest organ of the integumentary system. Skin performs the role of protection and sensation and other functions, such as heat regulation, storage for lipids and water, excretion, absorption, and so on.

The skin is composed of three main layers, the epidermis, the dermis, and a sub-dermal layer, or hypodermis. The major cell types that comprise these layers, including keratinocytes, fibroblasts, melanocytes, and endothelial cells, express NOS and appear capable of releasing NO.

Nitric oxide (NO) is a multifunctional signaling molecule active in many tissues of the body. Recent progress has allowed the identification of the nitric oxide pathway in several cell types that reside in the skin, including keratinocytes, melanocytes, Langerhans cells, fibroblasts, and endothelial cells.

Keratinocytes account for about 90–95% of the cells in the epidermis. Most of the evidence now indicates that keratinocytes constitutively express nNOS. The fibroblasts are the most abundant cell type in the dermis, where their role is to produce the fibrous extracellular matrix that gives the skin its mechanical resistance. Skin-derived fibroblasts have been shown to express NOS3 and in cytokine stimulation condition iNOS was also shown. The endothelial cells of normal human skin express eNOS in normal condition and express iNOS in the dermal endothelial cells of patients with atopic or allergic contact dermatitis.

In small controlled concentrations it acts as an intercellular signaling molecule exerting key regulatory and homeostatic functions in the everyday processes in normal human skin, such as vasodilation, melanogenesis and protective responses to environmental challenges. And NO in cutaneous biology is also involved in a wide range of pathophysiological processes throughout the skin for its cytotoxic and immunoregulatory properties.

Double-formula nitric oxide and epidermal growth

The in vitro experiments have shown that nitric oxide can cause the differentiation of proliferative keratinocytes. Additionally, nitric oxide can mediate the proliferation of endothelial cells resulting from the vascular endothelial growth factor (VEGF). By mobilizing different growth factors, nitric oxide can also help recovery. VEGF promotes the proliferation of vessels, which is the key factor for treating wounds, and is also achieved with the help of nitric oxide. The two complement each other: nitric oxide can promote keratinocytes to express VEGF and assists VEGF in stimulating proliferation of vessels, while VEGF in turn promotes the synthesis of nitric oxide by regulating the activity of NOS.

The concentration of NO is increased partially on skin to promote the growth of epidermal cells, without affecting the overall level of systemic nitric oxide.

Thus nitric oxide can improve wound healing, and the health of the skin.

NO gel or NO-derived cosmetics

NO is applied pharmacologically in various forms usually as NO donors to correct NO deficient state of to regulate the activities of many tissues. Topical application may be used to help wound and burn healing, hair growth and cause vasodilatation where needed.

Nitric oxide is effective in many kind of skin cells, and is associated with processes that deal with skin inflammation, immune skin disease and skin cancer. By promoting the synthesis of fibroblasts, nitric oxide can reduce pathological and physiological sequela in the early stages of inflammation and late stages of hyperplasis and during the tissue forming stage. Research has also shown that the NO synthesis of fibroblasts in hypertrophic scar tissues decreases. Nitric oxide can also affect the functions of langerhans cells, such as microbe extermination and the presentation of antigens to combat cellular viruses; it can also affect adjacent keratinocytes and melanocytes.

NO gel is our patented method for generating medically applicable nitric oxide. NO generated components are combined in a gel system (diffusion inhibiting medium) to control the rates of nitric oxide release and be sufficient viscous to topically apply.

Vasodilation

Nitric oxide dilates the blood vessels on the area where it is topically applied. The dilated blood vessels are able to carry more oxygen and nutrients needed for skin metabolism.

The constitutive release of NO by the endothelial cells of the microvasculature plays an important role in setting resting blood flow rate. Using laser-Doppler fluxmetry to measure blood flow, it was reported that the intradermal injection of the NOS inhibitor, L-NAME, significantly reduced flow rates in rat skin.

In conclusion, the constitutive release of NO in the skin is involved in setting the rate of resting blood flow, via a cGMP-dependent relaxation of the vascular smooth muscle.

Antimicrobiology

The idea that NO may serve as non-specific host defense has been aired since the early 1990s and it is now known that it exerts antimicrobial effects on diverse micro-organisms including fungi, yeast, bacteria, viruses, and protozoa.

Thus, as the front line against the invasion by pathogens, the constitutive and steady production of NO on the skin's surface is likely to play an important role.

Topically applied nitric oxide is a potentially useful preventive and therapeutic strategy against superficial skin infections, including MRSA infections.

Staphylococcus aureus is the most common gram-positive pathogens, can cause many kinds of human infection. Thus, with the widespread use of antibiotics, drug resistance problem is becoming more and more serious. In fact, humans' own innate immune system is effective to resist foreign microbial invasion as the first line of defense. One of the important mechanisms is induced nitric oxide synthetase system, the synthetic NO can direct inhibition MRSA aerobic energy metabolism and restrain DNA replication of MRSA, which plays a vital role in killing bacteria and pathogenic microorganisms.

Burn and wound healing

NO signaling appears to play a vital role in wound healing. NO involve in angiogenesis, mediating inflammatory process, cell proliferation and collagen disposition, then improving wound healing. The positive effects of arginine supplementation and NO donors, coupled to the negative effects of NOS inhibitors or the deletion of the NOS2 or NOS3 genes, have provided unassailable evidence of a key role for NO.

One of the key functions of NO in wound healing seems to be its permissive influence on keratinocyte and fibroblast proliferation, which helps promote wound re-epithelization.

The likely importance of NO-modulated cytokine signaling in the wound healing process seem to be the NO-induced activation of TGF-b1 and enhancement of IL-1 and IL-8 production. NO is also known to stimulate epithelial cells to produce and release chemokines and other growth mediators such as vascular endothelial growth factor (VEGF).

Our study used topical NO-gel on mice with second degree burn wounds, and found that the NO gel had the potential to enhance burn wound healing by regulation of many cellular processes in the skin. NO treatment promoted re-epithelization and wound closure by enhancing inflammatory cell infiltration, promoting angiogenesis, and facilitating collagen synthesis in the wound bed.

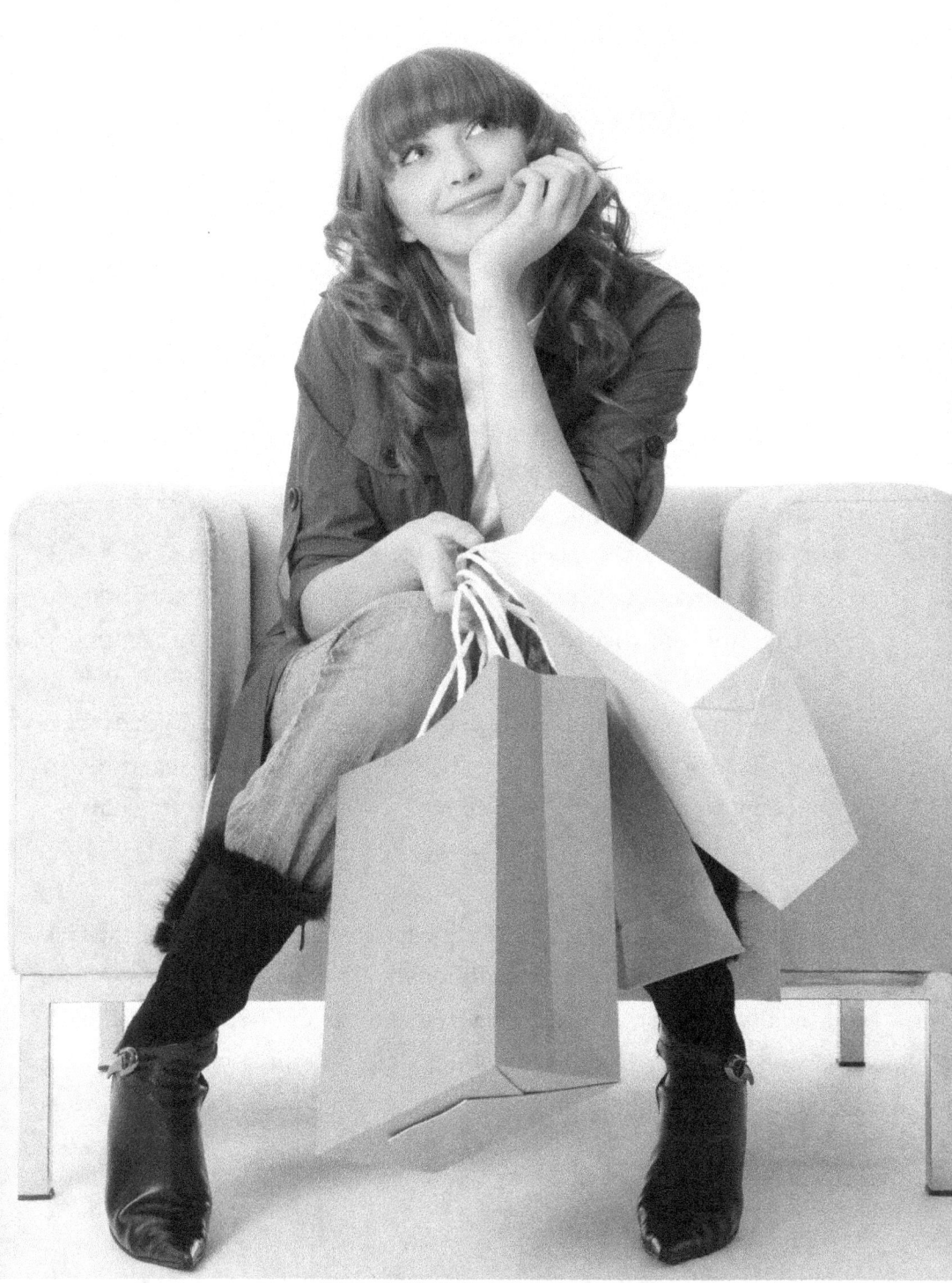

Chapter Seven
Obese Subjects as a Group

Obesity refers to a weight level to body size ratio that is significantly higher than normal and is due to an excessively thick fat layer. It occurs as a result of excessive accumulation of in vivo fat, especially triglyceride. Obesity can be categorized into two types: simple obesity and secondary obesity. In most cases, obesity refers to simple obesity: i.e., when weight exceeds the normal weight by over 20%.

Obesity not only affects work, life and appearance, but also is hazardous to health to some extent. The WHO has defined obesity as a disease that is the third major global health hazard in the developed world, alongside cardio-cerebrovascular diseases and cancer. Obese subjects are highly vulnerable to hypertension, coronary heart disease, fatty liver, diabetes, hyperlipemia, gout and cholelithiasis.

As clinical tests show, most patients with simple obesity are observed with endocrine disorder, especially hyperinsulinemia, glucose tolerance abnormality, disorder of sex hormone levels, higher adrenal cortical hormones, and leptin increases. Teenage obesity may also easily lead to sexual impotence. Early treatment of obesity is of important significance for preventing the diseases mentioned above.

Hazards of obesity

1) Life quality declines, working capacity is affected, and the risk of injury increases. Obese individuals are prone to sweating, have difficulty coping with excessive heat and can easily become fatigued, as well as suffer from leg swelling, skin inflammation and varicose veins. Severely obese individuals are often slow in their movements

and walk with difficulty, and can experience palpitations and short breath when exercising. It is therefore difficult for obese individuals to live a normal life, and their condition can sometimes prevent them from working. Excessive fat in the human body will also affect the balance of in vivo sexual hormones. For males, this can lead to a decline in sexual function and even impotence. For females, it can lead to failure to conceive. Since obese subjects act and react slowly, they may suffer indirect injuries as a result of their condition because of a higher risk of accidents.

2) High risk of coronary heart disease, hypertension and even the "quintet of death". Obese subjects possess increased levels of fat tissue, causing rising levels of oxygen consumption and an increased burden on the heart, which can lead to cardiac hypertrophy. Over a long time, they may easily develop hypertension. Deposits of fat in the arterial walls can lead to luminal stenosis, sclerosis, coronary heart disease, and stroke. For this reason, obese individuals are highly vulnerable to the so-called "quintet of death", namely coronary heart disease, hypertension, hyperlipemia, diabetes (non-insulin-dependent) and cerebrovascular diseases. If an individual suffers from all five of these conditions, it is important to take swift action to avoid fatality.

3) Harmful effects on pulmonary function. Pulmonary function refers to the supply of oxygen to the whole system and the release of CO_2. Due to increased weight, obese subjects require more oxygen, but the lungs cannot increase their function to provide oxygen beyond a certain level. Additionally obese subjects possess large deposits of fat around the abdomen, causing pressure in the abdominal cavity to rise. This has the effect of pushing the diaphragm upwards and in turn causes pressure in the chest cavity to increase, thus restricting respiratory function of the lung and resulting in hypoxia. This causes

sleepiness, dyspnea, polycythemia, right ventricular hypertrophy, and eventually cardiac and pulmonary dysfunction. There is a special pulmonary heart disease, also known as ventilation syndrome or adverse pulmonary ventilation syndrome, also called Pickwickian syndrome, which if not promptly treated, has a fatality rate of up to 25%. Due to deposits of fat around the neck of obese subjects, this will result in periodic trachea occlusion during sleep, which may lead to insomnia, snoring, oxygen and sleep deprivation.

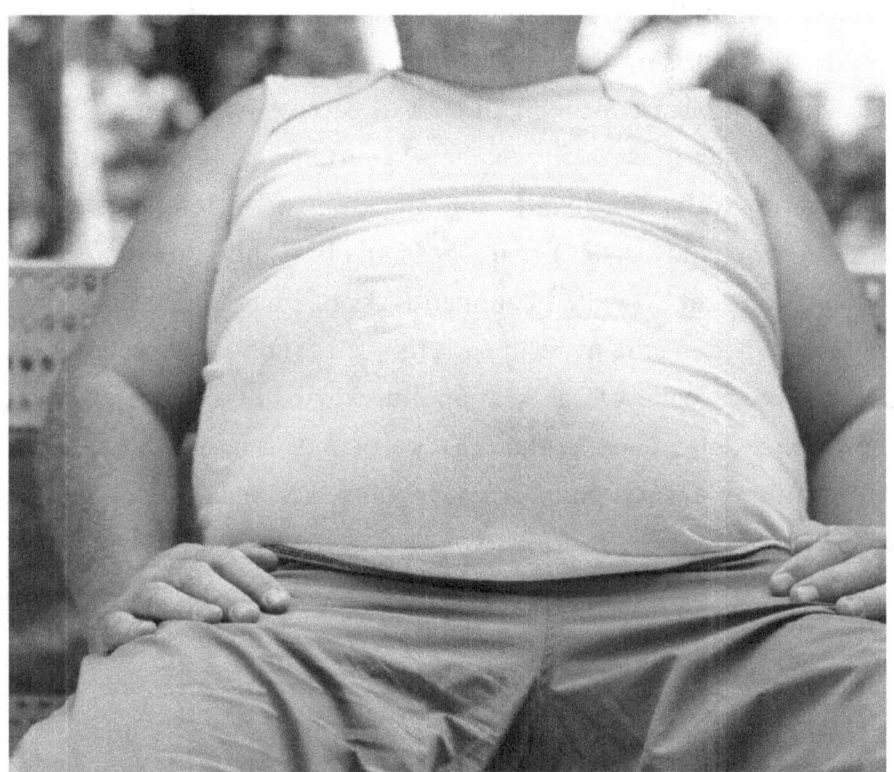

Nitric oxide shows a great effect on obesity subjects as a group

1) Nitric oxide can reduce the risk for obesity subjects of cardio-cerebrovascular diseases

Nitric oxide is an important factor for keeping blood flow smooth. By dilating vessels, clearing vascular inter wall attachments, repairing injured endothelium in vessels, and clearing blood refuse, it ensures that blood circulates properly throughout each of the body's organs. It can also help to remove refuse in the blood that accumulates as a result of obesity, and reduces the risk of different cardio-cerebrovascular diseases that are caused by obesity.

2) Nitric oxide can help obese subjects to improve their pulmonary function

By dilating pulmonary vessels, nitric oxide plays an important role in regulating the physiological and pathological process of pulmonary circulation. Therefore, exogenous nasal delivery of nitric oxide is of great importance for the treatment of different pulmonary hypertensions. As nitric oxide can be combined with hemoglobin to inactivate quickly, nasal delivery of nitric oxide is only effective on pulmonary vessels, but not in systemic circulation. Clinical research also proves that delivery of (20—40ppm) nitric oxide can significantly help obese subjects as a group to improve their pulmonary function.

Chapter Eight
Sexual Dysfunction

Sexual dysfunction refers to the failure to achieve a satisfactory level of sexual performance. Sexual dysfunction mostly occurs without any organic disorder, but it is due to psychological factors. Hence, it is often called sexual psychological dysfunction.

For males, sexual dysfunction means inability to perform sexually; for females, it indicates an inability to achieve sexual satisfaction. Sexual dysfunction can be categorized into four main types: (1) depressed sexual desire, represented by lack of continual and propagative sexual interest and inhibited sexual arousal; (2) depressed sexual excitement, represented by obstructed ejaculation of male or vaginal lubrication in the female, such as impotence and sexual frigidity; (3) sexual orgasm depression, whereby the male is able to achieve erection and the female shows normal sexual excitement, but sexual orgasm is not achieved, either because of male or female inability to achieve orgasm, or because of male premature ejaculation (4) other sexual dysfunctions. The psychological reasons for the types of sexual dysfunction outlined above are comparatively complicated, owing to the unique living situation, life experiences and psychological profile of each patient. In China, traditional families always avoid any talk related to sex, resulting in late sexual education. Obviously, this can have certain effects on the psychology of young people.

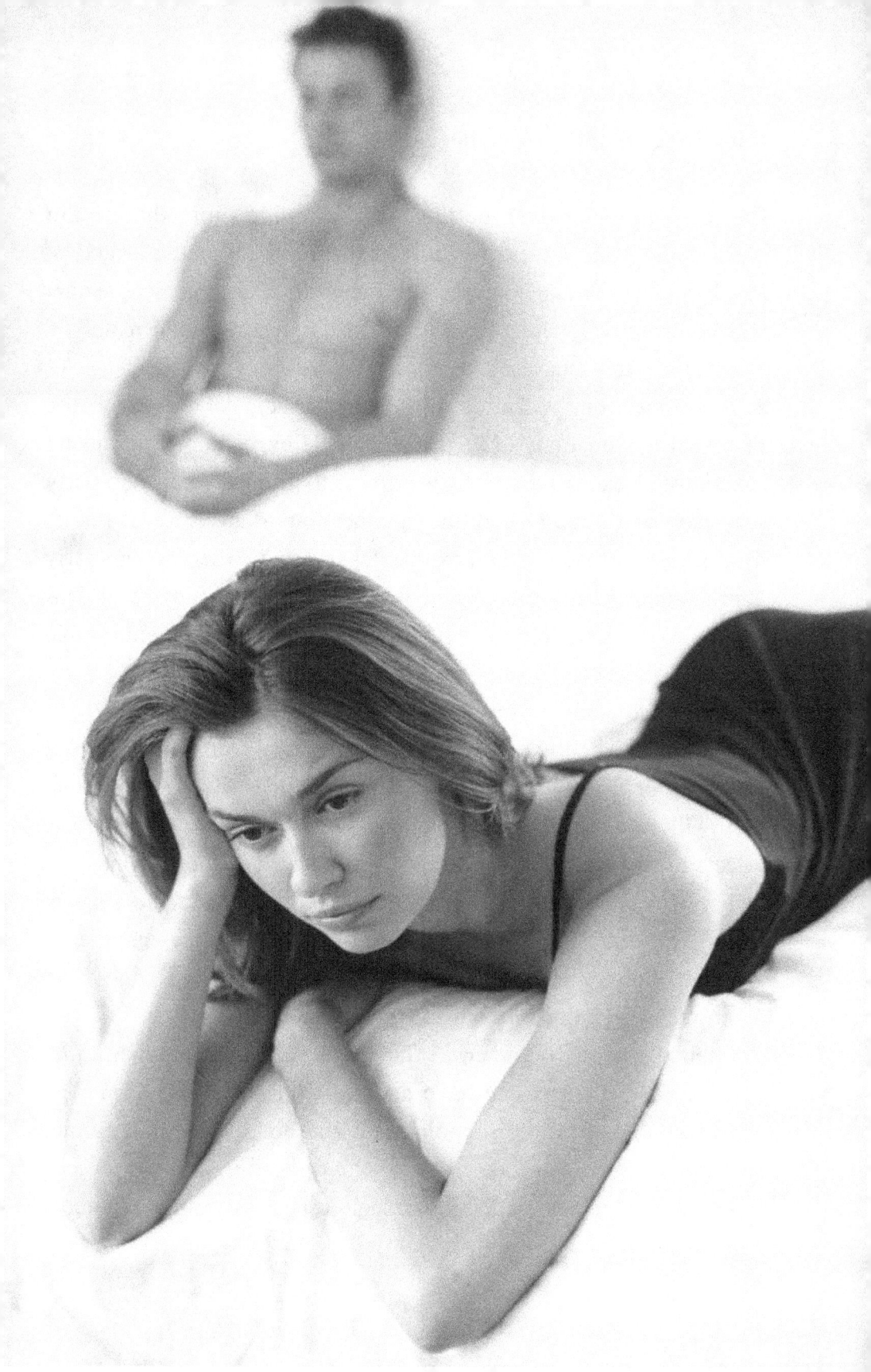

Causes for sexual dysfunction

Causes for sexual dysfunction may be divided into three main types: biological factors, psychological factors and cultural factors. Psychological factors are especially important. Psychological factors with comparatively direct impact on sexual function include mainly:

1) Attitudes towards sex

Sexual anxiety due to fear of failure may be the most common cause of sexual dysfunction, while the unrealistic expectations for sexual capability or excessive sexual requirements from the opposite party can also contribute. In addition, another important cause of sexual dysfunction is to act as an anxious "bystander", whereby one party attaches an extreme importance to the response of the other party. This can make it impossible for both parties to interact in a comfortable way.

2) Effect and conflict of past sexual experiences

If one person has experienced strict control, punishment, cruel treatment or injury in their past sex experiences, it is possible that they will still bear the psychological scars of this experience. The effects of these experiences are hard to eliminate from the memory and may even condition the response of the individual to subsequent sexual encounters, leading to sexual dysfunction such as impotence and lack of orgasm.

3) Impact of relationship tensions on sexual function

Personal tensions between sexual partners based on suspicion, jealousy and distrust can have an effect on sexual performance. Obviously, the strong disappointment and hostility of one partner will provoke the same response of the opposite party, which can have a highly negative effect on sexual desire. For example, females

242

are often very sensitive to the feeling of being "used", thinking the opposite party is only interested in her body and nothing more. This can be highly inhibiting for sexual arousal.

4) Psychological depression due to various external factors

Fast modern life, busy work, family matters, disharmonious personal relationships, competition and frustration at work, personal education background and social position all exert considerable psychological pressures on us in our daily lives. Needless to say, these psychological pressures can in turn have an effect on sexual function.

In addition to the above, sexual dysfunction is also affected by organic causes. In diagnosing sexual dysfunction, it is necessary to eliminate relevant physical diseases, such as chronic inflammation and injury of sexual organs and lesion of the relevant nervous system. Some endocrine diseases, the long-term use of some drugs, and mental diseases such as depression and anxiety neurosis may all result in sexual dysfunction.

5) Diabetic patients' sexual dysfunction

Over a long period of time, diabetes will result in sexual dysfunction to some extent, and some patients will even lose their sexual function. Diabetic sexual dysfunction is a special case: commonly used impotence drugs will not show any significant effects. The most common factors leading to diabetic sexual dysfunction include: Psychological behavior

It includes disharmony between spouses, anxiety, depression and other psychological factors. Over a long period of time, diabetic patients will develop problems such as physical fatigue, peripheral neuritis and perineural inflammation, all of which will affect the mood of patients and thus lead to an increase in sexual dysfunction. It is a psychological problem due to physiological reasons as well as a psychosomatic disease.

Recommendation: pay attention to your emotional state, participate in social activities and, if necessary, consult a psycho-therapist.

Inadequate hormone secretion

Diabetes is a form of endocrine disease, is considered by doctors to affects hormone secretion to an extent. According to some experts, to treat the inadequate secretion of sexual hormone secretion, use of impotence drugs stimulating secretion of sexual hormone secretion is effective, but this is not the case for diabetic patients. This indicates that there is not adequate evidence to explain inadequate secretion of sexual hormones among diabetics.

Recommendation: moderately increase intake of certain nutritional foods, such as wolfberry fruit, Chinese chive, onion and mutton.

Microangiopathy

Male and female genital organs contain abundant micro vessels. Over a long period of time, Diabetes causes metabolic function to decay gradually and it becomes possible to observe microangiopathy. This affects the hyperemia of genital blood organs and thus reduces sexual excitement. In turn, a decrease of sexual excitement over time will result in sexual dysfunction.

Recommendation: reduce entertainment, stop smoking or reduce smoking, avoid excessive drinking, control diet, increase the intake of cereals and if necessary, go to the doctor for assistance.

Injury of neural receptors

Because post-diabetic metabolic dysfunction causes injuries to neural receptors, this can also explain sexual dysfunction among diabetic patients, as sexual arousal is facilitated by the normal functioning of

244

the sensory organs.

Recommendation: take treatment as per therapy for diabetic complications.

Motion system reason

After suffering from diabetes for a long period of time, metabolic dysfunction results in insufficient muscular strength and physical weakness, which can also lead to sexual dysfunction. Recommendation: increase physical exercises.

Obviously, when use of impotence drugs for diabetic sexual dysfunction is not effective, metabolic function intervention techniques can also be used to improve micro circulation, repair neural receptors, and enhance the physical quality of patients. As practice proves, metabolic function intervention is of extreme importance to diabetic patients. As the sexual dysfunction attributable to diabetes is mostly secondary, it will be easier for this kind of objective therapy to show an effect.

Other reasons

(1) Relationship tensions between spouses, leading to declining sexual desire due to the antipathy towards the opposite partner.

(2) Excessively heavy working pressure may cause males to become physically fatigued and lose interest in any further physical activity, including sex.

(3) In Chinese culture, due to religious and educational factors, some middle-aged and elderly males may display unscientific prejudices towards sexual matters. It is believed by some that "one drop of

semen is equal to ten drops of blood", and that sexual activity can be highly damaging to one's health and thus should be avoided. Invariably, these attitudes can have a damaging effect on one's sex life

(4) Lack of communication between partners, common interests, mutual trust and involvement of discussion of problems can have a highly negative impact on people's sex lives.

(5) Undesirable living conditions, such as rooms that are not sound-proof or parent-child cohabitation.

(6) Sense of inferiority: feelings of weak sexual capability, poor physical condition, failure to achieve a satisfactory sexual life, preoccupation with personal afflictions and a sense of inferiority related to penis size can all lead to reduced sexual excitement.

(7) Extramarital affairs, gambling and prostitution, drug taking and excessive drinking, etc.

Prevention and treatment of male sexual dysfunction

In addition to psychological factors, for physiological or pathological prevention and therapy of male sexual dysfunction, it is critical to improve vein reflux in the corpus cavernosum, increase blood flow, and reduce intracavernous pressure. It is essential and fundamental for prevention and treatment of male sexual dysfunction that the integral vascular endothelium produces adequate nitric oxide and maintains blood flow through the cardio-cerebrovascular system. Sexual dysfunction is physiologically or pathologically related to the overall status of the human body and is a barometer of health in the human body. For any diseases that have the secondary effect of male sexual dysfunction such as hypertension and diabetes, prevention and treatment should be administered first, while in the meantime increasing the concentration of in vivo nitric oxide, taking moderate exercise, and increasing one's intake of food containing sufficient nitric oxide precursors or health-care foods containing antioxidants.

As living standards continue to rise in China, people's basic material needs can be met, allowing them to concentrate on the pursuit of further wealth and happiness. As an important part of happy family life, sexual life appears to be especially important. However, in real life, the fast pace of living and career pressure can cause many males to feel physically and mentally fatigued. Meanwhile, excessive smoking and drinking and other factors that promote male sexual dysfunctions, especially impotence and premature ejaculation, have recently displayed an upward trend.

NOS can modify the L-arginine molecule to generate nitric oxide and increase the release of in vivo nitric oxide. NOS is located in many cells including smooth muscle cells, neural fibers and endothelial cells, with corpus cavernosum containing the most and corpus spongiosum containing the least. Under sexual stimuli, NOS catalyzes the reaction of L-arginine and oxygen molecules to generate nitric oxide. Nitric oxide is a molecule with an extremely short half-life, and can quickly spread throughout the body to become combined with heme in guanylate cyclase to activate the enzyme so that guanosine triphosphate is transformed into cGMP. cGMP then stimulates cGMP-dependent protein kinase in vascular smooth muscle, so that vessels relax and dilate and blood flows into the corpus cavernosum for penile erection. Meanwhile, phosphodiesterase can degrade cGMP and can reduce the vascular smooth muscle relaxation effect of nitric oxide and cyclic GMP on the corpus cavernosum. Nitric oxide, cyclic GMP and phosphodiesterase are jointly involved in regulating the relaxation and contraction response of smooth muscle, fulfilling and maintaining penile erection. Drugs that inhibit phosphodiesterase are on the market for erectile dysfunction (ED) and enhance the effects of nitric oxide to increase cyclic GMP, thereby causing greater relaxation of the penile vessels and greater blood flow leading to erection.

Summary

This book shows us the relationship of nutritional supplements and diet with a very important messenger molecule in our body —— Nitric Oxide. One author of this book, Dr. Ferid Murad has researched Nitric Oxide over the past 35 to 40 years, and, for that work, he received the Nobel Prize in Physiology or Medicine in 1998. Another author of this book, Dr. Daniel Chen, was his closest student, aide and colleague. In this book, they summarize the importance of Nitric Oxide in a soft, understandable scientific way that the nonscientist would understand. They believe that understanding of Nitric Oxide can help people achieve a healthy lifestyle, and that a good understanding of nutritional supplements and diet will enable the readers to take a more proactive role in their health and hopefully in the prevention of some medical diseases.

PART ONE NITRIC OXIDE, A HEALTH MESSENGER

For many years, the public perception of Nitric Oxide was primarily negative, owing to the substance's reputation as an atmospheric pollutant released from car exhausts and refuse combustion. It wasn't until the 1980s that Ferid Murad, Robert. F. Furchgott and several other scientists were successful in determining the various health benefits of Nitric Oxide– and they made the important discovery of the function of Nitric Oxide in the vascular system. It was this ground-breaking discovery which was to throw new light on Nitric Oxide as an important "Health Messenger"; a discovery for which both Scientists received the Nobel Prize. The importance of Nitric Oxide in treating cardiovascular disease should by no means be underestimated, and new milestones in Nitric Oxide research are being reached each day.

PART TWO PURIFYING HEALTH AT THE SOURCE

We depend on the circulatory system not only to transport oxygen and life-giving substances to the various parts of our body, but also to discharge waste and refuse, constantly supplementing and purifying our bodies in a complete metabolic cycle. There is no doubt that blood and blood vessels are the keystones of human life and health. One might therefore ask: how can we ensure the health of this life giving system? What effect will vascular aging cause to health? What substances or processes are fundamental to the health of this system? Let us explore the processes on which we all depend to find the answers to these universally important questions.

PART THREE THE AMAZING PROPERTIES OF THE MIRACLE MOLECULE

Although state of mind, unlike the physical body, cannot be seen nor touched, it directly influences the amount of enzymes and activity of NOS in the body. Patients' psychological status influences their quality of life, and may also have a significant impact on their physical status, including cardiovascular health. The psychological status such as calmness of the mind raises nitric oxide levels in the human body, whilst anger and fear reduce nitric oxide levels. It is important to maintain a good psychological state to keep nitric oxide levels high; for longevity and enhanced quality of life.

PART FOUR "3A & 1S" HEALTHCARE METHODS TO LET YOU LIVE ANOTHER 30 YEARS

Nitric oxide can be acquired in such ways as food, moderate exercise and supplements of functional food, while appropriate supplements of antioxidants is another important method to keep nitric oxide formation increased. Therefore, the health-keeping method of "three acquisitions and one supplement" ensures adequate supply of nitric oxide for the body as well as avoids nitric oxide being removed due to rapid oxidation so that the body is always in a healthy state.

PART FIVE GROUPS IN NEED OF NITRIC OXIDE

As a kind of nutritional supplement, nitric oxide is involved in the circulation and metabolism of different systems in the human body and has an extremely important effect for health. What kinds of people need to supplement nitric oxide? As studies show, those who need to supplement include: elderly, mental workers, post-menopausal women, smokers as a group, alcohol drinkers as a group, obese subjects as a group and persons with hypothyroid. Obviously, these are large groups.